CLINICAL AND RESUSCITATIVE DATA

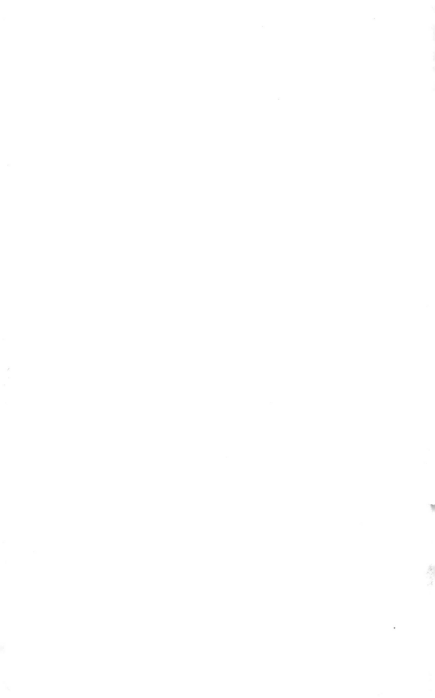

CLINICAL AND RESUSCITATIVE DATA

A Compendium of Intensive, Medical
and Anaesthetic Resuscitative Data

R.P.H. DUNNILL
MBBS FFARCS
Consultant Anaesthetist
Bournemouth and Poole Hospitals

M.P. COLVIN
BSc MBBS FFARCS
Consultant Anaesthetist
The London Hospital

THIRD EDITION

BLACKWELL SCIENTIFIC PUBLICATIONS
OXFORD LONDON EDINBURGH
BOSTON PALO ALTO MELBOURNE

© 1977, 1979, 1984 by
Blackwell Scientific Publications
Editorial offices:
Osney Mead, Oxford OX2 OEL
8 John Street, London WC1N 2ES
9 Forrest Road, Edinburgh EH1 2QH
52 Beacon Street, Boston
  Massachusetts 02108, USA
706 Cowper St, Palo Alto
  California 94301, USA
99 Barry Street, Carlton
  Victoria 3053, Australia

First published 1977
Second edition 1979
Third edition 1984

German edition by
Gustav Fischer Verlag 1983

Typeset by
Burns & Smith, Derby
Printed and bound in Great Britain
by Henry Ling Ltd, Dorchester

DISTRIBUTORS

USA
  Blackwell Mosby Book
  Distributors
  11830 Westline Industrial Drive
  St Louis, Missouri 63141

Canada
  Blackwell Mosby Book
  Distributors
  120 Melford Drive, Scarborough
  Ontario, M1B 2X4

Australia
  Blackwell Scientific Book
  Distributors
  31 Advantage Road, Highett
  Victoria 3190

British Library
Cataloguing in Publication Data

Dunnill, R.P.H.
  Clinical and resuscitative data.
  —3rd ed.
  1. Resuscitation—Handbooks,
      manuals, etc.
  I.   Title   II. Colvin, M.P.
  615.8'043   RO86.7

ISBN 0-632-01209-9

CONTENTS

Contents

Contents

Contents

PREFACE TO THIRD EDITION

The third edition of this book has been revised and improved in many ways. We have removed some of the more academic material and put in much more clinical information. This will be of greater relevance to practicing clinicians of all kinds.

The number of sections has been increased and in some cases extensively updated and revised. The introduction of an index should make the instant retrieval of information much easier.

Once again we would like to thank all those who took the trouble to inform us about mistakes in the Second Edition, and would be most grateful to those readers who tell us of any errors that may have crept into this one.

We would like to acknowledge and offer our thanks for the advice and help given to us in preparation of this edition to Dr Volans and his staff at the poisons centre, Guys Hospital, Dr Colin Blogg, Dr Ron Hill, Dr Andy Williams, Dr Jim Johnstone, and many others. Lastly we thank the patient staff of Blackwell Scientific Publications for their help and encouragement.

R.P.H. Dunnill
M.P. Colvin

PREFACE TO SECOND EDITION

In the second edition we have endeavoured to improve the formation and contents of this book, incorporating many of the suggestions and criticisms we have been grateful to receive.

The order of the items has been rearranged to help location of information, and some extraneous facts removed. Much had been added to the anaesthetic, paediatric and cardiac sections. We hope these improvements will make this edition even more useful than the first.

Our thanks go to Miss D. Barklay of the Dietetic Department, the London Hospital. To Dr Volans of the Poison Centre, Guy's Hospital, to Dr Jim Johnstone of the Biochemistry Department, Poole General Hospital, and to Dr Peter Green and Dr Brian Colvin for revising the haematology section.

R.P.H. Dunnill
M.P. Colvin

PREFACE TO FIRST EDITION

In practical and emergency situations there is often an urgent need for numerical data, formulae and general guidelines for treatment. It has been our purpose to provide this information in a logical and easy-to-find manner. This book is in no way a textbook or even a book on how to treat patients, it is a compendium of that data which is often hard to find but needed quickly in resuscitation procedures.

It is intended for all grades of junior staff in most specialities, especially those involved in accident and emergency departments, intensive care and other resuscitation areas.

The data comes from numerous sources and we have tried to include facts and formulae that will be safe to use and acceptable to most schools of thought. The book is arranged in sections and subsections, as shown in the list of contents. References are given at the foot of subsections and space is provided for personal notes and additions as new information and drugs come on to the market.

Whilst every effort has been made to ensure the accuracy of the information given, the authors would be grateful for any corrections as well as ideas for further inclusions.

We have in all cases endeavoured to trace and acknowledge the original source of material used. In addition we would like to thank the following for their kind help in producing this book: Dr Volans and Robin Braithwaite of Guy's Hospital, National Poisons Centre: Dr Sterndale, Consultant Haematologist; Mr Hoskins, Chief Pharmacist; Mr Stockhill, Chief Technician, Biochemistry Department; Mr D. Rodgers, Department of Medical Illustration, all at the Kent and Canterbury Hospital; Professor Strunin, Dr Ainley Walker, Dr Potter, Dr Wedley, for correcting the proofs; Mrs J. Atterbury and Mrs M. Allen for their secretarial help; and last but by no means least Blackwell Scientific Publications for their help and encouragement.

R. P. H. Dunnill
B. E. Crawley

SECTION 1
ACID BASE BALANCE

1.1 Siggard-Anderson alignment nomogram

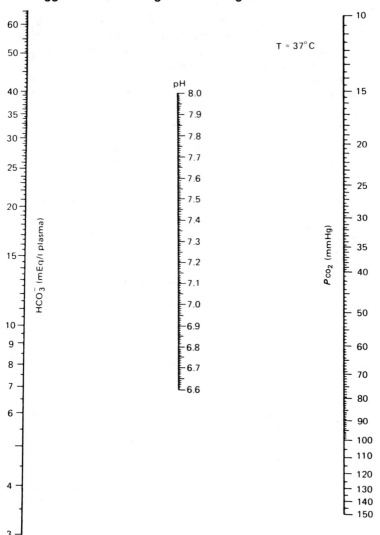

From the known pH and P_{CO_2} of the patient's blood gases the standard bicarbonate can be found by placing ruler across nomogram.

1.1.1 Temperature conversion table for pH and blood gases

Blood gas machines are maintained at a constant temperature of 37°C. If the patient's temperature differs from that of the machine, pH and blood gas results must be corrected, since the solubility of a gas in a liquid changes with temperature.

The following table, derived from a nomogram*, indicates the correction factors for the temperature difference. Since the effect of temperature on Po_2 varies with the haemoglobin saturation, figures are shown for low, normal and high ranges of uncorrected Po_2.

* Kelman G.R. & Nunn J.F. (1966) *Journal of Applied Physiology* **21**, 1484–90.

Patient temp.°C	kPa 33.2+ mmHg 250+ Multiply Po_2 by	12.2 92	5.99 45	Multiply Pco_2 by	Add to pH (pH units)
41	1.08	1.22	1.35	1.19	− 0.059
40	1.06	1.16	1.25	1.14	− 0.044
39	1.04	1.11	1.15	1.09	− 0.029
38	1.02	1.06	1.07	1.05	− 0.015
37	1.00	1.00	1.00	1.00	0.0
36	0.98	0.95	0.92	0.96	+ 0.015
35	0.96	0.91	0.86	0.92	+ 0.029
34	0.94	0.87	0.80	0.88	+ 0.044
33	0.92	0.84	0.75	0.84	+ 0.059
32	0.90	0.79	0.69	0.81	+ 0.074
31	0.88	0.75	0.64	0.77	+ 0.088
30	0.86	0.71	0.59	0.74	+ 0.103
29	0.85	0.68	0.56	0.71	+ 0.118
28	0.83	0.64	0.52	0.68	+ 0.132
27	0.81	0.61	0.47	0.65	+ 0.147
26	0.80	0.58	0.44	0.63	+ 0.162
25	0.78	0.56	0.41	0.59	+ 0.176

The top header spans: *Po_2 range* over the kPa/mmHg columns.

1.1.2   pH conversion table to nanomoles

pH units	H^+ nanomoles	pH units	H^+ nanomoles
3.0	1 000 000	6.0	1000.0
3.1	794 200	6.1	794.2
3.2	630 900	6.2	630.9
3.3	501 200	6.3	501.2
3.4	398 100	6.4	398.1
3.5	316 300	6.5	316.3
3.6	251 200	6.6	251.2
3.7	199 500	6.7	199.5
3.8	158 500	6.8	158.5
3.9	125 900	6.9	125.9
4.0	100 100	7.0	100.0
4.1	79 420	7.1	79.42
4.2	63 090	7.2	63.09
4.3	50 120	7.3	50.12
4.4	39 810	7.4	39.81
4.5	31 630	7.5	31.63
4.6	25 120	7.6	25.12
4.7	19 950	7.7	19.95
4.8	15 850	7.8	15.85
4.9	12 590	7.9	12.59
5.0	10 000	8.0	10.00
5.1	7942	8.1	7.942
5.2	6309	8.2	6.309
5.3	5012	8.3	5.012
5.4	3981	8.4	3.981
5.5	3163	8.5	3.163
5.6	2512	8.6	2.512
5.7	1995	8.7	1.995
5.8	1585	8.8	1.585
5.9	1259	8.9	1.259
6.0	1000	9.0	1.000

1.2   Acid base correction formulae

1.2.1   To correct metabolic acidosis

Give either
Base deficit x $\frac{1}{3}$ weight in kg ($\frac{1}{5}$ weight is more accurate in adults) as mmol sodium bicarbonate.
or
Base deficit x 20 x weight in kg as ml of THAM using a 0.3 molar solution.

The base deficit is the deficit of standard bicarbonate from the normal of 24.5 mmol/l.

1.2.2   To correct metabolic alkalosis in adults

Give either
250 mg Diamox 6 hourly until urine pH > 7 (2–6 hour delay before full effect).
or
Ammonium chloride 2 g t.d.s. orally.

As the pH falls by 0.1 unit the K^+ in plasma rises 0.6 mmol approx and vice versa.

1.2.3   To correct hyperkalaemia in adults

Give either
20 units of soluble insulin with 30 g of glucose
or
Na^+ Resonium or Ca^{++} Resonium 15 g t.d.s. orally or pr.

2

SECTION 2
**ANAESTHESIA
GENERAL AND
LOCAL**

2.1 Physical properties of anaesthetic gases and vapours

Name	Formula	Dates Discovered	Used	BP (°C)	Mol. wt.	Specific gravity Gas	Liquid
Carbon dioxide	CO_2	1757	1921	−78.5	44	1.50	1.2
Cyclopropane	$CH_2\,CH_2\,CH_2$	1822	1930	−33	42	1.46	0.58
Ethylene	$CH_2\,CH_2$	1779	1921	−104	28	0.97	0.34
Helium	He	1895		−269	4	0.18	0.13
Nitrogen	N_2	1772		−196	28	1.25	0.80
Nitrous oxide	N_2O	1772	1868	−88	44	1.53	1.2
Oxygen	O_2	1772	1794	−183	32	1.40	1.14
Chloroform	$CHCl_3$	1831	1847	61	119	4.10	1.47
Divinyl ether	$CH_2\,OCH_2$	1887	1932	28	70	2.20	0.78
Enflurane	$CHFClCF_2\,{-}O{-}CF_2H$	1965	1973	56	184.5	7.54	1.51
Ether	$C_2\,H_5\,OC_2\,H_5$	1540	1842	35	74	2.60	0.70
Ethyl chloride	$C_2\,H_5\,Cl$	1849	1894	13	64.5	2.3	0.9
Fluoroxene	$CF_3\,CH_2\,{-}O{-}CHCH_2$	1951	1953	43	126	4.4	1.1
Halothane	$CF_3\,CHClBr$	1951	1958	50	197	6.8	1.9
Isoflurane	$CF_3\,CHCl{-}O{-}CF_2\,H$	1965	1972	49	185	7.54	1.51
Methoxy- flurane	$CHCl_2.CF_2\,{-}O{-}CH_3$	1958	1960	105	165	5.7	1.4
Trichlor- ethylene	$CHCl.CCl_2$	1864	1934	87	131	4.40	1.47

BP = boiling point; SVP = saturated vapour pressure; MAC = minimum alveolar concentration. The concentration of anaesthetic agent required to produce lack of reflex response to a skin incision in 50% of subjects.
The specific gravity = relative density of the fluid to that of water (liquid) or in the case of a vapour to that of dry air (gases)

Sat. concn. = saturation concentration = $\dfrac{\text{SVP}}{\text{atmos press}}$ x 100

Specific volume = $\dfrac{\text{vol. vapour}}{\text{vol. liquid}}$

AD95 = Approaches to the theoretical minimum anaesthetic concentration by estimating the dose that anaesthetizes 95% of the population.

SVP mmHg (at 20°C)	AD95 (%)	MAC (%)	Flam. in O$_2$ %	Specific volume	Ostwald coefficients of solubilities at 37°C				approx. sat. concn.
					H$_2$O	Oil/Gas	Blood/Gas	Oil/H$_2$O	
42 200	–	–	0	–	55.5	–	–	–	–
4 800	10.1	10	2–60	300	0.20	11.5	0.45	39	650
–	74.5	65	2–80	272	0.09	1.3	0.41	–	–
–	–	–	0	–	–	–	–	–	–
–	–	–	0	–	1.2	–	–	–	–
39 760	–	101	0	400	0.44	1.4	0.47	2.2	5100
–	–	–	–	–	2.4	–	–	–	–
160	–	0.5	0	280	40	260	10	100	20
560	–	3.0	2–85	250	1.4	60	2.6	41.3	75
184	1.88	1.7	6	–	0.78	98	1.9	–	25
442	2.22	2.0	2–82	215	13	65	12	3.2	55
988	–	2.0	4–67	310	1.2	–	3.0	–	140
290	3.57	3.5	4	200	0.85	48	1.4	–	40
240	0.9	0.8	0	220	0.8	220	2.5	330	33
250	1.63	1.3	6	–	0.62	97	1.4	–	34
25	0.22	0.2	5–28	200	4.5	950	10.2	400	3
65	0.35	0.3	9–65	250	1.7	960	9.0	400	10

References

Atkinson R.S., Rushman G.B. & Lee J.A. (1982) *A Synopsis of Anaesthesia*. Wright, Bristol.
Churchill Davidson H. (1984) *A Practice of Anaesthesia*. Lloyd Luke, London.
de Jong R. H. & Eger E. I (1975) MAC expanded. AD50 and AD95 values of common inhalational anaesthetics in man. *Anaesthesiology* **42**, 384.
Eger E. I. *et al.* (1965) Minimum alveolar anaesthetic concentration: a standard of anaesthetic potency. *Anaesthesiology* **26**, 756.

2.2 Pressure and contents of gases in anaesthesia and medicine

Table indicates size of largest pin-indexed cylinders but larger cylinders with 'bull nose' or 'wheel' valves are available.

Gas	Colour code UK	USA	Filling pressure lbf/in²	kPa	Critical Press. (kPa)	Temp. (°C)	Largest pin index Size	Volume(l)
Oxygen	White top Black body	Green	1987	13 700	5079	-118.4	E	680
Nitrous oxide	Blue	Blue	638	4400	7260	36.5	E	1800
Entonox	White/blue top	–						
	Blue body	–	1987	13 700	–	–	G	5000
Carbon dioxide	Grey	Grey	725	5000	7380	31	E	1800
Cyclo-propane	Orange	Orange	65	500	5470	125	B	180
Helium	Brown	Brown	1987	13 700	2290	-268	D	300
Helium/ Oxygen 21%	White/ brown top black body	Brown/ green	1987	13 700	–	–	E	600
Ethylene	Purple	Red	1200	8268	5229	9.7	–	–
Air	White/black	Green/ white	1980	13 500	–	–	F	1280

The size and filling pressure data are for the United Kingdom, although those for the United States are similar.

2.3 Anaesthetic circuits

2.3.1   Minimum safe gas flows for anaesthetic circuits

Name of circuit	Minimum flow rates	
	Intermittent positive pressure ventilation	Spontaneous ventilation
Mapleson A		
Magill	2 x min vol.	min vol.
Lack	3 x min vol.	min vol.
Mapleson C		
Waters	3 x min vol.	2 x min vol.
Mapleson D		
Bain	3 x min vol.	2 x min vol.
Mapleson E		
Copes	3 x min vol.	2 x min vol.
Ayre's T (see section 2.3.2.)		
Circle System	$\frac{1}{3}$ min vol.	250 ml O_2

2.3.2   Ayre's T-piece system — see Mapleson E circuit (2.3.1)

Age	Fresh gas flow (l)	Reservoir limb (ml)	
0–3 months	3–4	6–12	
3–6 months	4–5	12–18	
6–12 months	5–6	18–24	or more
1–2 years	6–7	24–42	
2–4 years	7–8	42–60	

Ayre P. (1965) The T piece technique. *British Journal of Anaesthesia* **28**, 520.

2.4 Anaesthetic endotracheal tube and circuit data

2.4.1 Endotracheal tube size

Age (years)	Tube size		Length (cm)		Tracheostomy			Broncho-scope
	Magill	Int. diam. (mm)	Oral	Nasal	Int. (mm)	French Gauge	Ext. (mm)	
0–3 months	00	3.0	10	–	–	–	–	Suckling
	0A	3.5	10–11	–	–	–	–	
3–6 months	0	4.0	12	15	4.0	–	5.5	Infant
6–12 months	1	4.5	12	15	4.5	–	6	
2	2	5.0	13	16	5.0	21	7	
3	2	5.0	13	16	5.0	21		
4	3	5.5	14	17	5.5	24		Child
5	3	5.5	14	17	5.5	24		
6	4	6.0	15	18	6.0	27	8	
7	4	6.0	15	18	6.0	27		
8	5	6.5	16	19	6.5	28	8.5	Adolescent
9	5	6.5	16	19	6.5	29		
10	6	7.0	17	20	7.0	30	9	
11	6	7.0	17	20	7.0	30	9	Small
12	7	7.5	18	21	7.5	32	10	adult
13	7	7.5	18	21	7.5	32	10	
14	8	8.0	21	24	8.0	33	11	
15	8	8.0	21	24	8.0	33		
16	8	8.0	21	24	8.0	33		Large
17	9	9.0	22	25	9.0	36	12	adult
18	9	9.0	22	25	9.0	36		
20	10	9.5	23	26	10.0	39	13	
22	10+	10.0+	23	26	11.0+	42	14	

Below 8–10 years, non-cuffed tubes should be used.

2.4.2 Endotracheal tube size formulae

The following formulae give rule of thumb methods of assessing tube size, tube lengths, etc., with an accuracy of $\pm 10\%$.

2

1 Tube size $= \dfrac{\text{Age (yrs)}}{4} + 4.5$ mm

2 Oral length $= 12 + \dfrac{\text{Age (yrs)}}{2}$ cm

3 Nasal length $= 15 + \dfrac{\text{Age (yrs)}}{2}$ cm

4 Dead space $= 2$ ml/kg or 1 ml/lb

5 Tidal volume $= 3 \times$ dead space or 7–10 ml/kg above 10 kg weight.

Reference

Atkinson R.S., Rushman G.B. & Lee J.A. (1982) *A Synopsis of Anaesthesia.* Wright, Bristol.

2.5 Drugs in anaesthesia

2.5.1 Premedication in children

It is usual to give anaesthetic drugs to children according to their body weight. The paediatric prescribing regimen from the section on drugs is also repeated here as another rough guide to drug doses in children.

Paediatric prescribing regimen

Age	Average wt (kg)	Proportion of adult dose (%)
2 months	3.2	10
4 months	6.5	15
1 year	10	25
5 years	18	33
7 years	23	50
12 years	37	75
15 years	55	85
Adult	66	100

Anticholinergic drugs orally or i.m.

Weight (kg)	Atropine (mg)	Hyoscine (mg)	Glycopyrrolate (mg)
0–12	0.2	0.15	0.1
12–20	0.3	0.2	0.15
20–50	0.4	0.3	0.2
>50	0.6	0.4	0.4

Sedative and analgesic drugs

Drug	Dose	Route
Vallergan Forte	2–4 mg/kg	o.
Omnopon	0.3 mg/kg	i.m.
Pethidine	1 mg/kg	i.m.
Phenergan	0.4 mg/kg	i.m.

These drugs are those most commonly used in children. Doses of other drugs are shown in the next section.

2.5.2 Anaesthetic infusion doses

All based on approximately one m.i.r. (minimum infusion rate).

	on air	on 60% N$_2$O
Althesin	35 μg/kg/min	18 μg/kg/min
Althesin +	24 μg/kg/min	16 μg/kg/min
	+	+
Alfentanil	0.4 μg/kg/min	0.25 μg/kg/min
Etomidate	37 μg/kg/min	23 μg/kg/min
	with 0.1 μg/kg/min Fentanyl	
Methohexitone	60 μg/kg/min	

2.5.3 Premedication and general anaesthetic drugs and doses

Non-proprietary name	Adult dose	Paediatric dose
Anaesthetic induction drugs		
Alphaxalone + alphadolone	3 ml i.v.	0.05 ml/kg
Etomidate	20 mg i.v.	0.3 mg/kg
Ketamine	500 mg i.m.	8 mg/kg i.m.
	150 mg i.v.	2 mg/kg i.v.
Methohexitone	100 mg i.v.	1.5 mg/kg
Propanidid	500 mg i.v.	7.5 mg/kg
Thiopentone	300 mg i.v.	4.5 mg/kg
Analgesics		
Alfentanil	0.25-1 mg i.v.	15-50 μg/kg i.v.
Buprenorphine	0.2–0.4 mg sub.ling	
	0.3–0.6 mg i.m.	Not in children
Diamorphine	5 mg o., i.m., i.v.	
	Extradural: 2–5 mg in 10 ml saline	–
Fentanyl	50–100 μg i.m.	1–3 μg/kg i.v.
	50–250 μg i.v.	
Fentanyl 50 μg/ml + Droperidol 2.5 μg/ml	1–2 ml i.m.	0.4–1.5 ml i.m. for
	Induction: 6–8 ml	premed.
	Maintain: 1–2 ml	
Methadone	5–10 mg o., i.m., i.v.	–
Morphine	10–15 mg i.m.,	0.2 mg/kg i.m.
	5 mg i.v.	0.1 mg/kg i.v.
	Extradural and intrathecal: 2–4 mg preservative free morphine in 10 ml saline	
Papaveretum	20 mg i.m. 4 h	0.4 mg/kg i.m.
	2.5 mg i.v.	
Pentazocine	30–60 mg s.c., i.m., i.v.	Max 1 mg/kg i.m.
		0.5 mg/kg i.v.
	50 mg 4 h o.	6–12 yr: 25 mg 4 h o.
Pethidine	50–100 mg i.m. 4 h	1 mg/kg i.m. 4 h
	10–20 mg i.v.	
	50–150 mg 4 h o.	0.5–2 mg/kg o.
Phenoperidine	1–2 mg i.v.	0.1–0.15 mg/kg i.v.

Doses of other analgesic drugs can be found in the pharmacology section (p.142).

Non-proprietary name	Adult dose	Paediatric dose
Anticholinergic drugs		
Atropine	Premed 0.6 mg i.m.	see previous section (p.14)
	Reversal of relaxants	0.02 mg/kg i.v.
	1-2 mg i.v.	
Glycopyrrolate	0.2-0.4 mg i.m., i.v.	0.004-0.008 mg/kg i.m., i.v.
	Relaxant reversal: Adults and children 0.01 mg/kg with 0.05 mg/kg Neostigmine	
Hyoscine	0.4 mg i.m.	see previous section (p.14)
Propantheline	30 mg i.v.	–
Anticholinesterase drugs		
Neostigmine	2.5 mg i.v.	0.05 mg/kg
Tetrahydroamino-acridine (THA)	15 mg i.v.	Not applicable
Antiemetic drugs		
Domperidone	10-20 mg o., i.m., i.v.	0.2-0.4 mg/kg o., i.m.
Droperidol	5 mg i.m.	0.3 mg/kg i.m.
Metoclopramide	5-10 mg o., i.m., i.v.	1 mg o., i.m., i.v.
		3-5 yr:2 mg
		6-14 yr:2.5 mg
Perphenazine	4 mg t.d.s. o.	
	5 mg i.m. 6 h	Not in children
Prochlorperazine	12.5 mg i.m.	–
Thiethylperazine	10 mg t.d.s. o.	
	6.5 mg i.m.	
	6.5 mg rectally	Not in children
Drugs in deliberate hypotension		
Diazoxide	300 mg i.v. rapidly	5 mg/kg i.v.
Hydralazine	20 mg i.v. slowly	–
Labetalol	10-20 mg i.v. repeat depending on effect, or infusion 1 mg/ml	–
Nitroprusside	50 mg in 500 ml 5% Dextrose	–
	Max. 400 μg/min. Use drip counter and burette.	
Pentolinium	Up to 10 mg in 0.5 mg increments	–
Phentolamine	Up to 10 mg i.v. in 1 mg increments.	–
	Infusion: 10 mg in 100 ml adjust rate for effect	
Trimetaphan	250 mg in 500 ml 5% Dextrose.	
	Infuse according to response	

2

17

Non-proprietary name	Adult dose	Paediatric dose
Muscle relaxant drugs		
(a) Depolarising		
Decamethonium	3-5 mg i.v.	0.05 mg/kg
Suxamethonium bromide or chloride	75–100 mg i.v.	1 mg/kg

(b) Non-depolarising (for children under 6 months half the paediatric dose should be used.)

Alcuronium	15–20 mg i.v.	0.25 mg/kg
Atracurium	0.3–0.6 mg/kg	0.3–0.6 mg/kg
Fazadinium	75 mg i.v.	0.9 mg/kg
Gallamine	120 mg i.v.	1.5 mg/kg
Pancuronium	6 mg i.v.	0.07 mg/kg
Tubocurarine	35 mg i.v.	0.4 mg/kg
Vecuronium	0.08–0.1 mg/kg	Not in children
Narcotic antagonists		
Nalorphine	5 mg i.v.	0.1 mg/kg
Naloxone	0.1–0.2 mg i.m. i.v.	1.5–3 μg/kg Neonates: 0.01 mg/kg
Levallorphan	1–2 mg i.v. i.m.	0.25 mg < 6/52 1 mg 1–5 years 2 mg > 5 years
Sedatives and premedicants		
Amylobarbitone	200 mg o.	–
Chloral hydrate	1–2 g o.	30–50 mg/kg o.
Chlorpromazine	25–50 mg o. 25–50 mg i.m. 5–10 mg i.v.	Over 5 yr: $\frac{1}{3}$–$\frac{1}{2}$ adult dose o, i.m. Under 5 yr: 5–10 mg o, i.m.
Diazepam	5–10 mg o, i.m., i.v.	0.1 mg/kg
Droperidol	5–10 mg i.m., i.v. 5–20 mg o.	0.2–0.3 mg/kg i.v. 0.3–0.6 mg/kg i.m. 0.2–0.6 mg/kg o.
Haloperidol	5 mg i.m., o.	–
Lorazepam	2–4 mg o. 0.025–0.5 mg/kg i.m., i.v.	Not in children
Midazolam	0.07 mg/kg i.v., i.m.	–
Pentobarbitone	100–200 mg o.	Not in children
Promazine	50 mg i.m. 25–100 mg o.	Proportional to adult dose on weight basis.
Promethazine	25–50 mg o., i.m.	–
Quinalbarbitone	200–300 mg o.	50–100 mg o.
Temazepam	10–30 mg o.	–
Trimeprazine	3–4.5 mg/kg o.	2–4 mg/kg o.
Vasoconstrictor drugs		
Ephedrine	Up to 10 mg i.v. 10–30 mg i.m.	– –
Metaraminol	1 mg i.v., 5 mg i.m.	–
Methoxamine	5 mg i.m., i.v.	–

2.5.4 Treatment of malignant hyperpyrexia

This condition in susceptible individuals exposed to a precipitating drug, is characterized by a rapid rise in temperature to very high levels during general anaesthesia. There may be a family history of death during anaesthesia.

Signs and symptoms

Rapid rise in temperature, muscle rigidity, tachycardia, tachypnoea, cyanosis, dysrhythmia. Myoglobinuria, acute renal failure, failure of coagulation.

Laboratory findings

Hyperkalaemia, hypoxia, hypercarbia, hyperphosphataemia, hypocalcaemia. Clotting screen may demonstrate disseminated intravascular coagulation (DIC)

Treatment

As soon as this condition is suspected:
1 discontinue anaesthesia and surgery;
2 inflate lungs with 100% oxygen through a clean circuit;
3 start surface cooling;
4 give Dantrolene 1 mg/kg i.v. at 5–10 min intervals to a total of 10 mg/kg;
5 correct potassium with glucose and insulin intravenously;
6 give methyl prednisolone 30 mg/kg;
7 correct acidosis with sodium bicarbonate or THAM;
8 give an initial dose of mannitol 20%, 20 g or 100 ml;
9 if DIC develops, consult a haematologist.

Drugs in anaesthesia

Possible precipitating factors

Halothane, enflurane, fluoroxene, methoxyflurane, trichloroethylene, diethyl ether, chloroform, cyclopropane
Tubocurarine, gallamine
Suxamethonium

Probable safe drugs

Regional blockade
Thiopentone, althesin, ketamine
Nitrous oxide
Pancuronium
Fentanyl
Droperidol
Promethazine

2.5.5 Antacids in obstetric anaesthesia

Obstetric patients undergoing elective or emergency procedures, whether in labour or not, should be protected as far as possible from the dangers of inhalation of stomach contents. An attempt should be made to reduce the volume of stomach contents and increase their pH above 2.5.

There is evidence that magnesium trisilicate may itself cause lung damage, and the following regimen is suggested.

Patients in labour:
Oral administration of 0.3 molar sodium citrate 30 ml, 15 min before anaesthesia.

If labour has been particularly prolonged, and the patient has received pethidine, consideration should be given to emptying the stomach and giving sodium citrate before induction of anaesthesia.

Elective obstetric procedures:
Cimetidine 400 mg orally nocte and cimetidine 400 mg i.m. 90 min before anaesthesia. Sodium citrate 30 ml can also be given 15 min before anaesthesia.

References

Cohen S.E. (1979) Aspiration syndromes in pregnancy. *Anesthesiology* **51**, 375–7.
Lahiri S.K., Thomas T.A. & Hodgson R.M.H. (1973) Single dose antacid therapy for the prevention of Mendelson's syndrome. *Brit.J.Anaes.* **45**, 1143.
Gibbs C.P., Spohr L. & Schmidt D. (1982) The effectiveness of sodium citrate as an antacid. *Anesthesiology* **57**, 44–6.

2.6 Local anaesthetics

2.6.1 Local anaesthetic drugs and doses

Pharmacological name (and proprietary)	Amount supplied (%)	Maximum adult dose without adrenaline (mg)	Onset time (min)	Duration (h)	Spinal solution	Epidural solution (%)
Bupivacaine (Marcain)	0.25–0.5	150	15–45	3–6	2 ml 0.5%	0.25–0.5
Cinchocaine (Nupercaine)	0.02–0.1	75	5–15	3–4	4 ml 0.5%	–
Cocaine	4–10	100 (topical only)	–	–	–	–
Etidocaine (Duranest)	0.5–1	300	6–10	5–7	–	1
Mepivacaine (Carbocaine)	0.5–2	200–300	5–15	$1\frac{1}{4}$–3	2 ml 4%	1–2
Prilocaine (Citanest)	1–2	400–600	5–15	3–5	2 ml 4%	1–2
Procaine (Novocaine)	0.5–2	700–1000	5–15	$\frac{3}{4}$–$1\frac{1}{2}$	4 ml 5%	2
Tetracaine/amethocaine (Pontocaine)	0.05–0.25	150–200	15–45	$3\frac{1}{2}$–6	2 ml 1%	0.25
Lignocaine (Xylocaine)	0.5–1.5	150–200	5–15	$1\frac{1}{4}$–3	4 ml 4%	1–2

Side effects

1 Cardiac
   a Myocardial depression
   b Bradycardia

2 Central nervous system
   a Excitation — convulsion
   b Inhibition — coma

3 Anaphylaxis
   a Rash
   b Hypotension
   c Bronchospasm

Treatment of side effects

1 Cardiac
   a Atropine 0.6 mg
   b Isoprenaline 4 μg i.v. (see section **4.2.1**)
   c Oxygen

2 Central nervous system
   a Anticonvulsants, diazepam 10–20 mg i.v.
   b Intubation and ventilation
   c Fluids
   d Oxygen

3 Anaphylaxis
   a Aminophylline 250 mg i.v.
   b Adrenaline 0.5 mg s.c.
   c Fluids
   d Intubation and ventilation
   e Oxygen
   f Hydrocortisone 200 mg i.v.

2.6.2   Dermatomes: the whole body

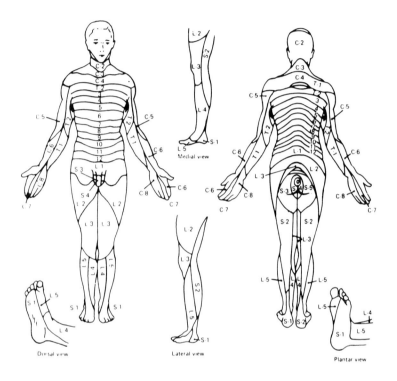

Dermatomes of the body representing segmental distribution of spinal nerves according to classical teachings, based on Foerster's data.

From **Bonica J. J.** (1953) *The Management of Pain.* Henry Kimpton, London. Reproduced by courtesy of author and publisher.

2.6.3 Dermatomes: the limbs

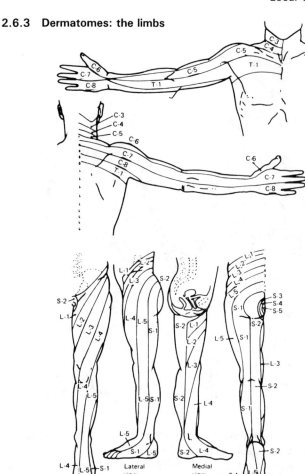

Dermatomes of the limbs as determined by the pattern of hypoalgesia from loss of a single nerve root.

From **Keegan J. J.** (1947) *Arch. Surg.* **55,** 246. Reproduced by courtesy of the publisher.

2.6.4 Sclerotomes

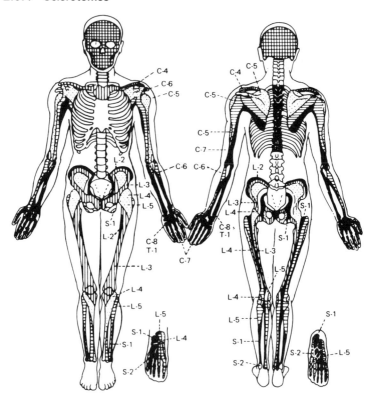

The various patterns moderate the fields of supply of each spinal segment. The skull is innervated by the trigeminal nerve and posterior primary rami of C_2; the vertebrae by the posterior divisions of the respective spinal nerves, and the ribs by both posterior and anterior primary divisions of the respective spinal nerves. The insets show the sclerotomes of the feet.

From **Bonica J.J.** (1953) *The Management of Pain.* Henry Kimpton, London. Reproduced by courtesy of author and publisher.

2.6.5 Innervation of the viscera: summary of the anatomy of visceral pain

Structure	Pathway	Entrance into central nervous system	Location of pain
Meninges of the brain	5th, 9th, 10th, 12th cranial nerves	Sensory nuclei in medulla	Frontal, temporal, parietal and/or over orbital region
Eye	Ophthalmic branch of the trigeminal nerve	Sensory nucleus of trigeminal in medulla	Orbit and frontal region
Lacrimal gland	Facial and glossopharyngeal nerves	Nucleus of tractus solitarius in medulla	Orbit
Parotid gland	Auriculotemporal branch of trigeminal – facial and glossopharyngeal nerves	Nucleus of tractus solitarius in medulla	Parotid region
Submaxillary and sublingual glands	Lingual nerve – facial nerve geniculate ganglion	Nucleus of tractus solitarius in medulla	Submaxillary region
Thyroid gland and capsule	Along sympathetics; cervical spinal nerves	T-1, T-2, C-2 to C-4	Anterior portion of the neck
Larynx	Superior and recurrent laryngeal nerves	Medulla	Throat and anterior neck
Trachea and bronchi	Along upper thoracic sympathetics; vagus	T-2 to T-7 Medulla	Sternal region
Lung parenchyma	Insensitive		
Parietal pleura	Intercostal Brachial plexus Phrenic nerve	T-1 to T-12 C-8, T-1 C-3 to C-5	Over affected portion Supraclavicular region Shoulder region
Heart	Middle and inferior cervical ganglia and thoracic cardiac nerves	T-1 to T-4 T-5*	Praecordium, left and sometimes right arm and chest

Structure	Pathway	Entrance into central nervous system	Location of pain
Thoracic aorta	Sympathetics	T-1 to T-5 or 6	Upper left chest and neck
Abdominal aorta	Sympathetics	T-6 to L-2	Lower chest, abdominal wall
Oesophagus	Inferior cervical sympathetic nerve; thoracic cardiac sympathetic nerves	T-5, 6, 7, 8	Midsternal region
Stomach	Greater splanchnic nerves; coeliac ganglia	T-6*, 7, 8, (9)	Epigastrium; interscapular region
Liver and gallbladder	Splanchnic nerves; coeliac ganglia	T-5*, 6, 7, 8, 9*	Right hypochondrium
Pancreas	Splanchnic nerves; coeliac ganglia	T-6, 7, 8, 10	Epigastrium; middle of back (T–10 and 11 vertebrae)
Spleen	Splanchnic nerves; coeliac ganglia	T-6, 7, 8	Left hypochondrium
Small intestine	Splanchnic nerves; coeliac ganglia	Duodenum, T-6, 7, 8 Jejunum and ileum, T-9, 10, 11	Epigastrium, umbilicus
Caecum; ascending and transverse colon	Splanchnic nerves and coeliac ganglia; lumbar sympathetic nerves	T-9, 10, 11	Suprapubic area
Appendix	Splanchnic nerves; coeliac ganglia	T-10, 11, 12 L-1	Right lower quandrant
Descending colon; sigmoid colon; rectum	Lumbar sympathetic nerves; aortic plexus parasympathetic nerves	L-1, 2 S-2, 3, 4	Deep pelvis Anus
Adrenal	Splanchnic nerves	T-10 to L-1	Loin
Kidney	Renal plexus; splanchnic nerves; upper lumbar rami	T-10, 11, 12 L-1, 2	Loin and groin

28

Ureters	Renal plexus; splanchnic nerves; upper lumbar rami	T-11,12	Loin and groin
Urinary bladder	Fundus – hypogastric plexus	L-1,2	
	Bladder neck – pelvic nerves and plexus	T-11, 12, L-1	Suprapubic region
Testes	Sympathetics	S-2, 3, 4	Perineum and penis
Prostate	Sympathetics	T-10	Testes
	Parasympathetics	T-10, 11	Perineum, low back
		S-2, 3, 4	
Uterus;	Body-sympathetics;	T-10, 11, 12, L-1	Lower abdomen; lower back
vagina	Cervix-pelvic nerves and pudendal plexus	T-11, 12, S-2, 3, 4	
perineum			Perineum
Ovary	Ovarian plexus – renal plexus – coeliac plexus	T-10	
Upper extremity	Brachial plexus	Somatic C-5, to T-1	Lower quadrants
Lower extremity	Lumbosacral plexus	Somatic L-4 to S-3	Affected segment } see 2.6.3. Affected segment }

*These segments inconstant

Reference

Bonica J. J. (1953) *The Management of Pain*. Kimpton, London.

2.6.6 Male genitourinary nerve supply

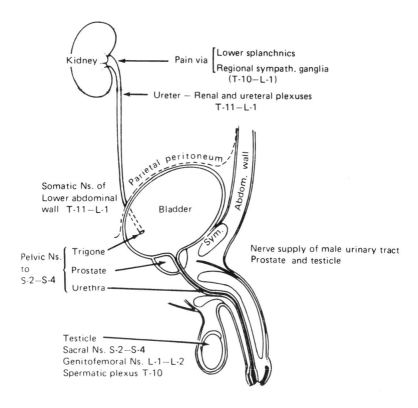

Kidney

Pain via [Lower splanchnics
Regional sympath. ganglia
(T-10—L-1)

Ureter — Renal and ureteral plexuses
T-11—L-1

Parietal peritoneum

Abdom. wall

Somatic Ns. of
Lower abdominal
wall T-11—L-1

Bladder

Sym.

Pelvic Ns.
to
S-2—S-4 { Trigone
Prostate
Urethra

Nerve supply of male urinary tract
Prostate and testicle

Testicle
Sacral Ns. S-2—S-4
Genitofemoral Ns. L-1—L-2
Spermatic plexus T-10

2.6.7   Female genitourinary nerve supply

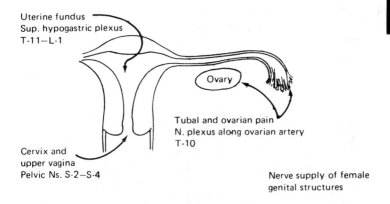

Uterine fundus
Sup. hypogastric plexus
T-11—L-1

Ovary

Tubal and ovarian pain
N. plexus along ovarian artery
T-10

Cervix and
upper vagina
Pelvic Ns. S-2—S-4

Nerve supply of female
genital structures

Adapted from **White J.C. (1943)** *Proc. A. Research Nerv. & Ment. Dis.* **23**, 373. With permission of publisher.

2.6.8 Types of block and local anaesthetic doses

This is not a text on technique, merely a dose reminder. The total dose is given when two or more injections are required to complete the block.

Block	Needle	Dose
Retrobulbar eye	2–3 cm 23 g	2% Lignocaine + adrenaline. + 150 units hyaluronidase.3 ml
Tonsillar	Spinal 22 g	1% Lignocaine + adrenaline. 30 ml total
I.V. Bier	Butterfly or similar 23 g	0.5% Lignocaine *plain*. 40 ml arm, 60 ml leg
Digital	2–3 cm 23 g	1% Lignocaine *plain*.1.5 ml total
Inguinal	2–3 cm 23 g	1% Lignocaine + adrenaline. 15 ml lat. 15 ml 10 med. 40 ml total
Penile	2–3 cm 23 g	1% Lignocaine *plain*.15 ml total
Gasserian ganglion	Spinal 22 g	2% Lignocaine 2 ml
Ophthalmic nerve	2–3 cm 23 g	2% Lignocaine + adrenaline. 2 ml
Maxillary nerve	2–3 cm 23 g	2% Lignocaine + adrenaline. 3 ml
Mandibular nerve	2–3 cm 23–25 g	2% Lignocaine + adrenaline. 5 ml
Mental nerve	2–3 cm 23–25 g	2% Lignocaine + adrenaline. 2 ml
Cervical plexus	Spinal 22 g	1% Lignocaine + adrenaline. 5 ml at each level
Brachial Plexus	3–5 cm 21 g	1% Lignocaine + adrenaline. 5 ml at each, 45 ml total
Ulnar, median, radial	2–3 cm 23 g	1% Lignocaine + adrenaline.5 ml each
Intercostal	2–3 cm 23 g	1% Lignocaine + adrenaline. 15 ml at each level
Paracervical	Special protected needle	1% Lignocaine + adrenaline. 15 ml each side
Pudendal	Spinal 22 g	1% Lignocaine + adrenaline. 15 ml each side
Sciatic	Sympathetic	1% Lignocaine + adrenaline.20 ml
Femoral nerve	Spinal 22 g	1% Lignocaine + adrenaline.20 ml
Obturator nerve	Spinal 22 g	1% Lignocaine + adrenaline.10 ml
Saphenous nerve	2–3 cm 23 g	1% Lignocaine + adrenaline.10 ml
Ankle	2–3 cm 23 g	1% Lignocaine *plain*.5 ml at the four sites, 20 ml total

Spinal	Spinal 22 g	4% Mepivicaine or Cinchocaine. 1-1.5 ml with positioning
Lumbar epidural	Epidural	1% Lignocaine *plain*. 15-30 ml 0.5% Bupivacaine *plain*. 8-15 ml
Thoracic epidural	Epidural	1% Lignocaine *plain*. 5-10 ml 0.5% Bupivacaine *plain*. 2.5-8 ml
Caudal epidural	3-5 cm 21 g	1% Lignocaine *plain* or 0.5% Bupivacaine. 10-35 ml
Stellate ganglion	Spinal 22 g	1% Lignocaine *plain* or 0.5% Bupivacaine *plain*. 5-10 ml
Lumbar sympathetic	Sympathetic	1% Lignocaine *plain*. or 0.5% Bupivacaine *plain*. 5-15 ml
Coeliac ganglion	Sympathetic	1% Lignocaine with adrenaline or 0.5% Bupivacaine. 25-20 ml

The spinal type needles have stilettes and are approximately 7-8 cm 20-22 gauge. The sympathetic type needles have stilettes and are approximately 15-17 cm 18-20 gauge.

We have used Lignocaine and Bupivacaine in these examples; for doses of other drugs see 2.6.1.

3.1 Rule of nines for determining area of burns

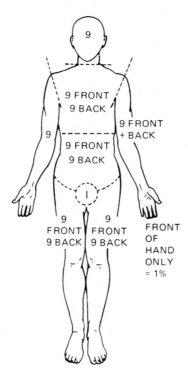

Figures represent percentage body area and add up to 100%.

Correction for head and neck and legs in children: subtract age in years from 12. Then:

1 for head and neck *add* result to the adult figure of 9% for head and neck, i.e. 5-year-old = 16%

2 for legs *subtract* the result from the adult figure of 36% for the legs, i.e. 5-year-old = 29%

3.2 Treatment of burns

3.2.1 Fluid requirements
1 Leeds method

$$\frac{\text{Total \% area of burns} \times \text{weight in kg}}{2} \text{ ml}$$

Give this volume of colloid for *each* of the following periods:

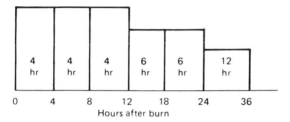

2 Alternative method based on Scandinavian method

A Colloid solution   1 ml × % total burn × wt (kg)
B Crystalloid   1 ml × % total burn × wt (kg)
C +1000 or more to make up total metabolic water requirements
if needed

1st day of burn 2A + B + C − ($\frac{1}{2}$ in first 8 hours and $\frac{1}{2}$ in next 16
hours)
2nd day $\frac{1}{2}$A + $\frac{1}{2}$B + C
3rd day $\frac{1}{2}$A + $\frac{1}{2}$B + C

The colloid can be plasma, dextran, Haemaccel or blood. The PCV
should be kept around 35%.
   Each 1% area of deep burn usually requires 1% blood volume
given as blood (see section 4.4.).
   In addition the normal metabolic water requirement should be
given (section 4.10). The electrolytes and osmolality should be
controlled as indicated by the serum and urine values.

3 Alternative Parkland method used in the USA

First 24 hours. Total fluid to be given = 4 ml × wt (kg) × % area burn (give $\frac{1}{2}$ the total in 1st 8 hours, $\frac{1}{4}$ the total in 2nd 8 hours and $\frac{1}{4}$ the total in 3rd 8 hours).

Use Hartmann's solution only; give blood if evidence of blood loss; monitor CVP.

3

Second 24 hours. Give 5% Dextrose in water plus sodium chloride, potassium to maintain electrolytes and replace other fluid losses, to maintain urinary output.

3.2.2 Other considerations

Urine output

Insert catheter. Output should be 0.5—1.0 ml/kg/hour. Give mannitol 0.75—1.0 g/kg if oliguria or haemoglobinuria, is present.

Analgesia

Adequate analgesia is always needed often in large doses to avoid systematic effects of severe pain. Morphine, papaveretum or pethidine are indicated. Satisfactory pain relief may be gained by continuous infusion of these drugs.

Respiratory

Burned patients may have inhaled chemical irritants, steam, or super-heated air. Frequent monitoring of respiration, clinical and biochemical status is needed to anticipate deterioration.

Alimentary

Nasogastric tubes should be inserted to prevent acute dilatation of the stomach, antacids should be given to prevent stress ulcers. As soon as gastric motility returns calories and high protein diet should be given by this route. Until then parenteral nutrition should be commenced with the normal regimen with additional 1 g/kg protein and 30 Cal/kg. Blood sugar must be monitored carefully.

Infections

During initial resuscitation in a non specialist unit, patient should be nursed in as clean an area as possible, such as ITU side room, or post operative recovery ward.

References

Muir and Barclay (1974) *Burns and their treatment.* Lloyd-Luke, London.
Evans A.J. (1975) *British Journal of Hospital Medicine* **13**, 287.
Boswick J.A., Thompson J.D. et al (1977) *Anaesthesiology* **47**, 164–70.

SECTION 4
CARDIAC FUNCTION

4

4.1 Cardiac data

4.1.1 Distribution of cardiac output to body organs

	Average wt (kg)	% body weight	Blood flow (ml/min)	% Cardiac output	O_2 consumption (ml/min/organ)
Brain	1.4	2.0	775	15	46
Heart	0.3	0.43	175	3.3	23
Kidneys	0.3	0.43	1100	23	18
Liver	1.5	2.1	1400	29	66
Lungs	1.0	1.5	175	3.5	5
Muscle	27.8	39.7	1000	19	64
Rest	38.7	55.34	375	9.7	33

4.1.2 Adult-neonatal cardiac comparison

	Adult	Neonate
Cardiac output	5 l/min	900 ml/min
O_2 consumption (ml/kg/min)	3.5	7.0
Blood pressure (mmHg)	120	45–75

4.1.3 Cardiovascular pressures

	Systolic (mmHg)	Diastolic (mmHg)	Mean (mmHg)
Peripheral venous	–	–	6–12
Right atrium(CVP)	–	–	0–7
Right ventricle	14–32	0–7	12–17
Pulmonary artery	14–32	2–13	8–19
Wedge or Left atrium	–	–	6–12
Left ventricle	100–150	2–12	
Arterial	100–150	60–90	80–100

4.2 Cardiac drug dilutions

4.2.1 Infusion rates for diluted drugs acting on the cardiovascular system

Infusion rates for dilutions other than those shown, can readily be calculated by appropriate multiplication or division.

	Drops/min	Microdrip 60 drops/ml	Standard 20 drops/ml	Other 10 drops/ml
1 mg/100 ml	1	0.2 μg	0.6 μg	1 μg
= 10 μg/ml	2	0.3	0.9	2
	5	0.8	2.4	5
	10	2	6	10
	20	3	9	20
	40	7	21	40
	60	10	30	60
	80	13	39	80
	100	17	51	100
10 mg/100 ml	1	2 μg	6 μg	10 μg
= 100 μg/ml	2	3	9	20
	5	8	24	50
	10	17	51	100
	20	33	99	200
	40	67	201	400
	60	100	300	600
	80	133	399	800
	100	167	501	1000

4.2.2 The usual dilutions of drugs used on the cardiovascular system by infusion

Diluent is 5% dextrose in all cases. In the interests of economy and safety it is usual to use a microdrip set incorporating a 100 ml burette to which the active drug can be added.

1 Adrenaline 1 mg in 100 ml. (1 ml of 1:1000 = 1 mg, 10 ml of 1:10000 = 1 mg)

2 Dobutamine 50 mg in 100 ml

3 Dopamine 200 mg in 100 ml

4 Isoprenaline 1 mg in 100 ml

5 Isosorbide 20 mg in 100 ml

6 Lignocaine 100 mg in 100 ml

7 Nitroprusside 50 mg in 100 ml

8 Noradrenaline 1 mg in 100 ml

9 Phentolamine 10 mg in 100 ml

10 Prenalterol neat infusion of 0.5 mg/min. Presented in 5 ml ampoules of 1 mg/ml

11 Salbutamol 1 mg (1 ml) in 100 ml

12 Glyceryl trinitrate (Tridil) 50 mg in 100 ml. Tridil and isosorbide are compatible with glass and polyethylene, but not with PVC containers. The containers made by Boots (Polyfusor), Dylade, Cheshire, and Antigen, Ireland, are all suitable.

Higher concentrations can be used if fluid restriction is necessary, or more effect is needed. The use of a drip counter with these drugs is mandatory.

4.2.3 Alternative dilution for dopamine and dobutamine

In some instances it is useful to be able to read the dose of an infused drug from the drip counter. This method applies to dopamine and dobutamine.

Multiply the body weight of the patient by 6. This gives the number of milligrams of the drug to be dissolved in 100 ml 5% dextrose. Make up this solution in the burette of a microdrip set (60 drops/ml). The setting of the drip counter now reads as the dose of the drug in μg/kg/min.

4.2.4 Drugs used in cardiovascular disease

Drug	Adult dose	Paediatric dose
Acebutolol	200 mg bd o. Initially. 5-25 mg i.v. slowly	
Acetazolamide	250 mg 6 h o., i.m., i.v.	Infant: 125 mg/day Child: 125-750 mg/day DD o.
Adrenaline 1/1000	0.5 mg = 0.5 ml s.c. 1 mg in 100 ml = 10 µg/ml by i.v. infusion	
Amiloride	5-20 mg daily o.	Not in children
Aminophylline	100-300 mg o. 360 mg b.d. rect. 250 mg i.v. slowly Infusion: 250 mg in 500 ml 6 h i.v.	Age Oral Rectal 0- 1 yr: 10-25 mg 12.5-25 mg b.d. 1- 5 yr: 25-50 mg 50-100 mg b.d. 6-12 yr: 50-100 mg 100-200 mg b.d.
Amiodarone	200 mg t.d.s. o. 150 mg i.v. slowly 5 mg/kg i.v. infusion over 30 min in 250 ml 5% dextrose	
Aspirin	300 mg daily o. anticoagulation	
Atenolol	50-100 mg daily o. 2.5 mg i.v. slowly (max. 10 mg in 20 min)	
Atropine	0.15 mg/kg i.v. infusion in 20 min 12 h 0.3-1 mg i.m., i.v.	0.02 mg/kg i.m., i.v.
Bendrofluazide	2.5-10 mg daily o.	—
Bethanidine	10 mg t.d.s. o.	—
Bretylium	5 mg/kg i.m. Repeat 6-8 h	—
Bumetanide	1-2 mg i.m., i.v. 1 mg daily o.	—

Drug	Adult dose	Paediatric dose
Calcium chloride	2.5-5 mmol i.v.	—
Captopril	25 mg t.d.s. o. Initially	—
Chlorothiazide	500 mg–2 g daily o.	—
Chlorpromazine	25–50 mg i.m.	—
	5–10 mg i.v.	
Chlorthalidone	50–100 mg daily o.	Up to 10 kg: 5 mg/kg alt. day o.
		Up to 5 yr: 50 mg alt. day o
		Over 5 yr; 50–100 mg alt. day o.
Clofibrate	Over 65 kg: 500 mg q.d.s. o.	—
	Under 65 kg: 500 mg t.d.s. o.	—
Clonidine	0.05–0.1 mg t.d.s. o. Initially	—
	0.15–0.3 mg i.v. slowly	—
Cyclopenthiazide	0.25–0.5 mg daily o.	—
Debrisoquine	10–20 mg daily or b.d. o.	Not in children
Diazoxide	300 mg i.v. rapidly	5 mg/kg i.v.
Digoxin	0.25–0.5 mg daily o., i.m.	0.01–0.02 mg/kg, repeat in 6 h then
		daily
Dipyridamole	Load dose: 0.5–1 mg i.m., i.v.,	
	repeat after 4 h	
Disopyramide	100-200 mg t.d.s. o.	5 mg/kg/day DD
	100 mg 6 h o.	
	2 mg/kg i.v. slowly. Max. 150 mg	
	Infusion: 0.4 mg/kg/h.	
	Max. 800 mg/24 h	
Dobutamine	Infusion: 50 mg in 100 ml.	
	Rate depends on effect	

Drug	Adult dose	Paediatric dose
Dopamine	Infusion: 200 mg in 100 ml. Rate depends on effect. Usually 5–10 µg/kg/min	
Ethacrynic acid	50 mg daily o., i.v. Initially	Over 2 yr: 25 mg daily o. Not parenteral
Frusemide	20–80 mg o., i.m., i.v.	1–3 mg/kg o. 0.5–1.5 mg/kg i.m., i.v.
Furosemide	See Frusemide.	
Glyceryl trinitrate	GTN tablets 1 p.r.n. sub. ling. Sustac: 2.5 mg t.d.s. Initially Nitrolingual: Metered oral spray o. Percutol: 1–2 ins 4 h percut. Tridil i.v. see section 4.2.2.	—
Guanethidine	20 mg daily o. 2–10 mg i.m.	—
Heparin	Load: 5000 units i.v. 10 000 units 6 h by infusion or by i.v. injection. Thromb. prophylaxis: 5000 units s.c. 12 h	
Hydralazine	25 mg b.d., t.d.s. o. 20–40 mg i.v. slowly	—
Hydrochlorothiazide	50–100 mg daily. Initially	—

Drug	Adult dose	Paediatric dose
Indoramin	25 mg b.d. o. Initially.	–
Isoprenaline	Sustained release: 30 mg 8 h o. Stat. i.v. dose: 10–20μg Infusion i.v: 1 mg in 100 ml or higher concn	–
Isosorbide	5–10 mg sub.ling. 10-30 mg q.d.s. o. Infusion: 2–10 mg/h i.v.	Not in children
Labetalol	100–200 mg b.d. o. 10–20 mg i.v. repeat depending on effect. Infusion: 1 mg/ml. Rate depends on effect	
Lanatoside C	Load dose: 0.8–1.6 mg i.m., i.v. over 24 h 0.25–1.5 mg/day o.	0.02–0.04 mg/kg i.v. then 0.01–0.03 mg/kg/day 3 DD o.
Lignocaine	100 mg i.v. stat. Infusion: 1–2 mg/min i.v.	–
Mecamylamine	2.5 mg b.d. o. Initially	–
Metaraminol	5 mg i.m., 1 mg i.v.	–
Methoxamine	5 mg i.m., i.v.	–
Methyldopa	250 mg b.d. t.d.s. o. Initially 250-500 mg 6 h i.v.	10 mg/kg/day 2–4 DD o. 20–40 mg/kg/day 4 DD i.v.
Metoprolol	50 mg b.d. o. Initially 5 mg i.v. slowly. Repeat up to 15 mg	–

4

49

Drug	Adult dose	Paediatric dose
Mexilitene	Load: 400 mg. Then 200 mg t.d.s., q.d.s. o. 100–250 mg i.v. slowly Infusion: 250 mg in 500 ml 0.5 mg (1 ml)/min	—
Minoxidil	5 mg daily o. Initially	0.2 mg/kg/day o. Max. 1 mg/kg/day
Nadolol	Angina: 40 mg/day o. Initially Hyperten: 80 mg/day o.	
Neostigmine	0.5 mg i.v. up to 2.5 mg	—
Nifedipine	10–20 mg t.d.s. o.	—
Nitroprusside	Recommended infusion: 50 mg in 500 ml 5% dextrose. A concentration of 50 mg in 100 ml may be necessary if fluid restriction required. Use drip counter and 100 ml burette. *Monitor carefully*	
Noradrenaline	1 mg in 100 ml 5% dextrose. Rate depends on response	—
Ouabaine	0.25–0.5 mg i.v. slowly	—
Oxprenolol	Angina: 40–160 mg t.d.s. o. Hyperten: 80 mg b.d. o. 2 mg i.m., i.v. slowly. Up to 16 mg	—

4

Drug	Adult dose	Paediatric dose
Pentaerythritol	30-60 mg t.d.s. o.	—
Pentolinium	Up to 10 mg i.v. 0.5 mg increments	—
Phenindione	1st day: 200 mg o.	
	2nd day: 100 mg o.	
	Then adjust to PTI	
Phenoxybenzamine	10 mg b.d. o. Initially	1–2 mg/kg/day o.
	1 mg/kg i.v. Very slowly	1 mg/kg i.v. Very slowly
Phentolamine	Up to 10 mg i.v. in 1 mg increments	
	Infusion: 10 mg in 100 ml, adjust	—
	rate for effect	
Phenylephrine	100 µg i.v.	
	Infusion: 10 mg in 100 ml, adjust	—
	rate for effect	
Phenytoin	3.5–5 mg/kg i.v.	—
Pindolol	2.5–5 mg t.d.s. o.	—
Practolol	5–10 mg i.v.	—
Prazosin	0.5 mg b.d., t.d.s. o. Initially	—
Prenalterol	2.5 mg i.v. slowly.	
	Infusion: 0.5 mg/min	—
Procainamide	250 mg 6 h o.	
	25 mg/min i.v. Max. 1 g	
Propanolol	10–40 mg t.d.s. o.	0.25–1 mg/kg t.d.s. o.
	1–2 mg i.v.	0.025–0.1 mg/kg i.v.
Protamine	1 mg neutralises 1 mg (100 units)	—
	of heparin.	
	Usual dose 3 mg/kg	

Drug	Adult dose	Paediatric dose
Quinidine	200–400 mg b.d. o.	–
Salbutamol	Infusion 3–20 µg/min i.v.	–
Sotalol	80 mg b.d. o. Initially 10–20 mg i.v. slowly	–
Timolol	10 mg daily o.	–
Tocainide	400 mg t.d.s. o. 500–750 mg i.v. slowly, or infusion in 100 ml N saline in 20 min	–
Triamterene	150–250 mg/day o.	Not in children
Verapamil	40–120 mg t.d.s. o 10 mg i.v. slowly and repeat 5 mg Infusion: 5–10 mg/h. Max. 100 mg/24 h	–
Warfarin	10 mg, 5 mg, 5 mg on Day 1,2 and 3, then PTI to establish maintenance	–

4.3 ECG times

4.3.1 Normal ECG times

P wave	Atrial wave	<0.10 s
PR interval	Atrioventricular conduction	0.12–0.20 s
QRS time	Rapid ventricular depolarization	0.05–0.08 s
QT time	Length of ventricular complex	0.35–0.40 s
T wave	Repolarization	≤0.22 s

4.3.2 Calculating rate/min from the ECG trace at 25 mm/s

Small squares = 0.04 s
Large squares = 0.2 s   i.e. 5 small squares = 1 large square

If 1 large square lies between R waves = rate of 300/min
   2 large squares lie between R waves = rate of 150/min
   3 large squares lie between R waves = rate of 100/min
   4 large squares lie between R waves = rate of 75/min
   5 large squares lie between R waves = rate of 60/min
i.e. 300 divided by number of large squares between R
waves = pulse rate.

4.4 Arrhythmias and abnormal ECG patterns

Sinus bradycardia. Usually between 40-60 beats/min. PR interval
increased, QT interval increase.
Clinical significance. Can be normal (sleep) or due to high vagal
tone.
Treatment. Usually none. If symptomatic, atropine 0.6–1 mg i.v. or
consider pacing.

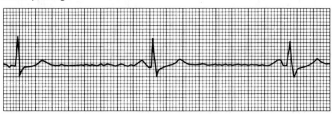

ECG times

Atrial fibrillation. Atrial rate if visible 400–700 beats/min, ventricular rate irregular often fast, up to 200 beats/min.
Clinical significance. Usually indicates heart disease.
Treatment. Patients with longstanding atrial fibrillation secondary to cardiac disease will usually be on digoxin. Acute atrial fibrillation can be treated by:
1 Verapamil 5–10 ml i.v. slowly. This drug must not be used if the patient is already taking beta blocking drugs.
2 Disopyramide 100 mg or 2 mg/kg (max. 150 mg) i.v. over 5 minutes.
The effect should last about 7 hours.
3 Digoxin 0.5 mg-1.0 mg followed by 0.25 mg b.d. i.m. then 0.25 mg daily.
4 DC shock.

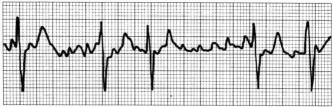

Atrial flutter. Atrial rate 200–400 beats/min with 2:1 or 3:1 ventricular response. Ventricular rate thus 100 to 150 beats/min. Flutter F waves visible.
Clinical significance. Ventricular rate needs to be controlled.
Treatment.
1 Verapamil 10 mg i.v.
2 Consider disopyramide 2 mg/kg i.v.
3 Consider practolol 5-10 mg i.v. NOT within 8 h of verapamil.
4 Consider DC shock.

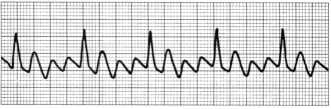

Figures on pp. 54–60 from the German edition (1983) by kind permission of Gustav Fischer Verlag, Stuttgart.

First degree atrioventricular block. PR interval greater than 0.20 s.
Clinical significance. Frequently none.
Treatment. None.

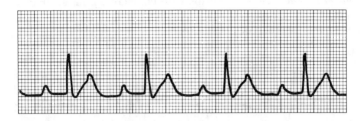

4

Second degree atrioventricular block. Usually 2:1 ratio of atrial to
ventricular beats. Rate about 40 beats/minute. PR interval constant
but prolonged.
Clinical singificance. May progress to third degree (complete) A–V
block and/or ventricular asystole.
Treatment. Usually none but 0.6–1 mg i.v. atropine may be tried.

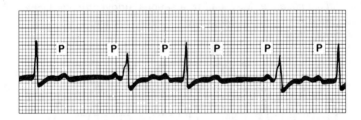

Third-degree block (complete). P waves occur regularly, but are dissociated from a variably deformed ventricular complex. The rate is usually slow.

Clinical significance. Grave if the QRS complex is bizarre. VF or asystole may supervene.

Treatment. Insertion of pacemaker.

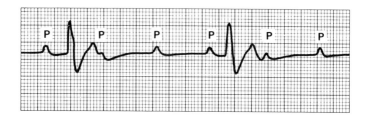

Left bundle branch block. Seen in leads V_1 or V_6. The broad-notched QRS complexes and deformed S-T segments are individually reminiscent of ventricular ectopic complexes.

Clinical significance. May lead to a serious atrioventricular block associated with significant ischaemic heart disease.

Treatment. None.

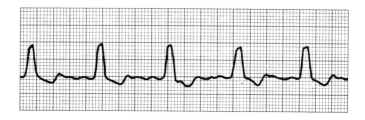

Right bundle branch block. Seen in leads aVr or V_1 as a typical RSR pattern, shown here with normal sinus rhythm. When these bizarre, wide, repetitive QRS complexes do not follow obvious P waves, they can be difficult to distinguish from those of ventricular tachycardia.

Clinical significance. May herald atrioventricular block if it follows cardiac infarction.

Treatment. Usually none, but if RBBB is associated with ECG evidence of left axis deviation and a long P-R interval, insertion of a temporary pacemaker should be considered.

4

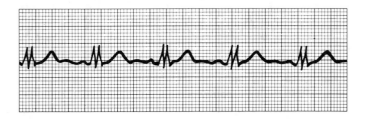

Pacemaker rhythm. It is common to see the pacing impulse just before an altered QRS complex but the pacing flash may be absent. P waves are not usually present but may occasionally be observed.

Clinical significance. Satisfactory capture of the heart rhythm by the pacemaker. When used in the 'demand' mode, the pacemaker may have some or all complexes suppressed by the patient's spontaneous complexes.

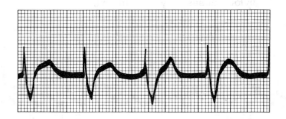

Atrial extrasystole. A normal P wave and QRS complex, but irregular rhythm. PR interval of extrasystole slightly shortened, or P wave within QRS complex.

Clinical significance. Essentially benign. May herald atrial tachycardia, flutter or fibrillation (AF).

Treatment. None.

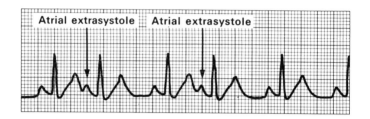

Supraventricular tachycardia. Normal QRS wth fast rate and P waves or within the QRS complex.

Clinical significance. May revert spontaneously but if prolonged or cardiac output is compromised treatment is necessary.

Treatment.

1 Carotid sinus pressure or Valsalva manoeuvre.

2 Verapamil 10 mg i.v. slowly. This dose can be repeated slowly after $\frac{1}{2}$ hour if necessary with frequent blood pressure monitoring.

3 Consider DC shock, particularly if the patient's condition deteriorates.

4 If there is no response 24 hours after verapamil, practolol up to 20 mg i.v. in divided doses may be effective.

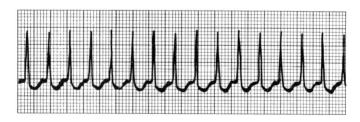

Ventricular extrasystoles. Abnormal ventricular extra beat occurs often, with abnormal T wave. No P wave precedes the abnormal beat.

Clinical significance. May precede ventricular tachycardia (VT) or ventricular fibrillation (VF)

Treatment. The decision whether to treat or to ignore ventricular extrasystoles depends on individual circumstances. These include the frequency of the abnormal beats their aetiology and the patient's general condition. Possible treatments include the following.

1 Lignocaine 100 mg i.v. If this is successful, a lignocaine infusion at a rate of 2 mg/min is the next step.

2 Check plasma potassium, blood sugar, blood gases and acid-base balance. Digoxin overdose may be an aetiological factor. A central venous pressure or Swan-Ganz catheter, or a mediastinal chest drain may all cause myocardial irritation.

3 Mexilitene 100–250 mg slowly i.v. Followed by an infusion of 1 mg/min.

4 Disopyramide 100 mg i.v. slowly. This can be followed by an infusion of 20–30 mg/h or 0.4 mg/kg/h to a maximum of 800 mg/day.

5 Phenytoin 3.5–5 mg/h i.v. is sometimes effective.

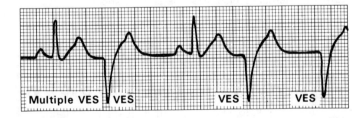

Multiple VES | VES | VES | VES

Ventricular tachycardia. Regular fast rhythm with abnormal ventricular complexes. Wide notch QRS complexes frequently seen. Rate usually 140–180 beats/min.
Clinical significance. Potentially dangerous except for 'slow' forms. High risk of transition to VF.
Treatment.
1 Lignocaine 100 mg i.v.
2 Disopyramide 100 mg i.v. slowly.
3 DC shock.

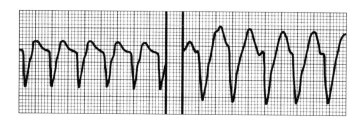

Ventricular fibrillation. Chaotic irregular ventricular pattern. However some semblance of QRS complexes may be seen.
Clinical significance. Circulatory arrest.
Treatment. External cardiac massage and DC shock.

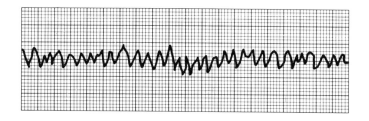

5.1 Normal blood values

Normal values tend to vary from laboratory to laboratory, depending on reagents and techniques used. We have taken these figures from many sources and the conversion factors are obtained from our own laboratory. If in doubt contact your own laboratory.

The second column contains the current units, followed by a conversion factor. The fourth column contains SI units where applicable, and the final column a symbol of the specimen of blood required and the amount in ml.

C	use a plain bottle for clotted sample
H	use a lithium heparin bottle for sample
B	use a heparinized blood sample (i.e. in a heparinized syringe)
EDTA	use a sequestrene bottle for sample.

In some cases the laboratory will collect the sample, and will supply special bottles.

5.1.1 Biochemistry normals

Name	Values in current units	Conversion factor	Values in SI units	Remarks
Acetone	0.3–2.0 mg%	172	51.6–344 μmol/l	H (5 ml)
Aldolase	0.9–2.5 iu/l	2.4	2.2–5.5 iu/l	C (10 ml)
Amino acid nitrogen	4–8 mg%	0.714	3–6 mmol/l	H (10 ml)
Ammonium	20–50 μg%	0.59	12–13 μmol/l	H (5 ml)
Amylase	80–180 Somogyi u%	0.375	70–30 iu/l	H (5 ml)
Arsenic	5–10 μg%	0.13	0.67–1.3 μmol/l	
Base excess	± 2 mEq/l	1	±2 mmol/l	H (5 ml)
Bicarbonate, actual	24–32 mEq/l	1	24–32 mmol/l	H (5 ml)
standard	21–25 mEq/l	1	21–25 mmol/l	
Bilirubin total	0.3–1.1 mg%	17.1	3–18 μmol/l	C (5 ml)
conjugated	<0.4 mg%	17.1	<7.0 μmol/l	C (5 ml)
Bromide	0.7–1.3 μg%	1	0.7–1.33 μmol/l	C (10 ml)
Bromsulphalein (BSP)	<5% after 45 min, giving			C (10 ml)
	5 mg/kg i.v.			
Buffer base	48 mEq/l	1	48 mmol/l (pH 7.4: P_{CO_2} 40)	H (15 ml)
Cadmium	0.3–0.5 μg%	0.09	0.027–0.045 μmol/l	C (15 ml)
Caeruloplasmin	30–60 mg%	0.25	300–600 mg/l	C (15 ml)
Calcium, total	8.5–10.5 mg% (4.5–5.7 mEq/l)	0.25	2.25–2.6 mmol/l	
ionized	4–5 mg%	0.25	1–1.25 mmol/l	C (15 ml)
Carbon dioxide P_vCO_2	40–52 mmHg	0.133	5.3–6.9 kPa	B (5 ml)
P_aCO_2	34–46 mmHg	0.133	4.5–6.1 kPa	B (5 ml)
content	48–52 ml%	1	48–52 ml%	H (10 ml)
Carotenoids	100–300 μg%	0.0186	1.8–5.5 μmol/l	
Catecholamines	1 μg%	54.6	<54.6 nmol/l	
Chloride	95–105 mEq/l	1	95–105 mmol/l	H (5 ml)
Cholesterol	140–300 mg%	0.026	3.6–7.8 mmol/l	H (6 ml) age dependent

5

5.1.1 Biochemistry normals *(continued)*

Name	Values in current units	Conversion factor	Values in SI units	Remarks
Cholinesterase, acetyl	—	—	9–25 μmol/ml/min	C (10 ml)
plasma	40–100 units%	—	—	C (10 ml)
Chromium	2–6 μg%			
Copper	80–150 μg%	0.157	13–24 nmol/l	EDTA (10 ml to poison centre)
Cobalt	0.3 μg%	169	50.7 nmol/l	C (10 ml)
Cortisol 0900 h	9–23 μg%	27.6	250–650 nmol/l	H (10 ml)
2400 h	<7.2 μg%	27.6	<200 nmol/l	H (10 ml)
	—	—	828 nmol/l	H (10 ml) neonatal cord blood
Creatine	0.2–0.8 mg%	76	15.2–60.8 μmol/l	H (10 ml)
Creatinephosphokinase	100 iu/l 60 iu/l	—	<60 iu/l ♂ <60 iu/l ♀	C (10 ml)
Creatinine	0.5–1.4 mg%	88.4	45–120 μmol/l	H (5 ml)
Fibrinogen	200–500 mg%	0.01	2.0–5.0 g/l	citrate bottle (10 ml) (lab. collects)
Folate	3–20 ng/ml	1	3–20 μg/l	C (10 ml)
Fluoride	0.014–0.019 mg%	528.6	7.4–10 μmol/l	C (10 ml)
Glucose, fasting	55–85 mg%	0.055	3.0–4.6 mmol/l	fluoride bottle (1 ml)
postprandial	<180 mg%	0.055	<10 mmol/l	C (10 ml)
γ-Glutamyl transferase	7–24 iu/l	2.2	10–55	fluoride bottle (1:5 ml)
Glycogen storage	Blood sugar >45 mg% over fasting level, 45 mins after subcut. inject. of epinephrine 0:01 mg/kg			
Gold	0.1–40 μg%			

2-hydroxybutyrate dehydrogenase (HBD)	50–130 iu%	10	500–1300 iu/l	C (10 ml)
Iodine total	3.5–8.0 µg%	78	273–624 nmol/l	C (10 ml)
Iodine 131 uptake	20–50% of administered dose in 24 h			C (10 ml)
Iron	80–160 µg%	0.179	14–30 µmol/l	C (10 ml)
Iron binding capacity	250–400 µg%	0.179	45–69 µmol/l	C (10 ml)
Isocitric dehydrogenase (ICD)	2–4 iu	10	20–140 iu/l	C (10 ml)
Ketones (as acetone)	0.8–1.4 mg%	98	80–140 µmol/l	H (10 ml)
Lactate	3.6–15 mg%	0.111	0.4–1.6 mmol/l	(lab. collects)
Lactic dehydrogenase (LDH)	100–300 iu		30–90 iu/l	C (5 ml)
Lead	10–40 µg%	0.0483	0.5–2.0 µmol/l	EDTA (10 ml)
Lipase	0–15 µ/ml			C (10 ml)
Lipids, total	400–1000 mg%	0.01	4.0–10.0 g/l	C (10 ml)
S particles	0.550 mg%	0.01	0–5.5 g/l	C (10 ml)
M particles	0–240 mg%	0.01	0–2.4 g/l	C (10 ml)
L particles	0–28 mg%	0.01	0–0.28 g/l	C (10 ml)
Magnesium	1.8–2.4 mg% 1.4–2.8 m Eq/l	0.411	0.7–1.00 mmol/l	C (5 ml)
Manganese	2.2 µg/l	18.2	40.0 nmol/l	C1 (15 ml)
Methaemoglobin	0.01–0.5 g%	10	0.1–5 g/l	EDTA (5 ml)
Mercury	0–5 µg%	0.05	0–0.25 µmol/l	(lab. collects)
Nicotinic Acid	0.0016–0.005 mg%	81.50	0.13–0.41 µmol/l	C (10 ml)
Nitrogen (non-protein)	18–30 mg%	0.714	12.8–21.4 mmol/l	C (10 ml)
Nickel	6.3 µg%	0.16	0–1.0 µmol/l	(lab. collects)
Noradrenaline	0.05 µg%	59	2.95 nmol/l	C (5 ml)
5-Nucleotidase	1.5–17 iu/l	1	1.5–17 iu/l	
Osmolality	280–300 mosmol/kg	1	280–300 mosmol/kg	H (15 ml)
pH venous	7.32–7.42		38–48 nmol/l	B (5 ml)
pH arterial	7.36–7.45	—	36–44 nmol/l (H^+ ion)	B (5 ml) arterial
P_{CO_2} arterial	34–46	—	4.5–6.1 kPa	B (5 ml) heparinized
P_{O_2}	90–110 mm Hg	0.133	12–15 kPa	B (5 ml)

5.1.1 Biochemistry normals *(Continued)*

Name	Values in current units	Conversion factor	Values in SI units	Remarks
Phenylalanine	1–3 mg%	0.061	0.06–0.2 mmol/l	H (5 ml)
Phosphate (inorganic)	2.0–4.5 mg%	0.323	0.64–1.4 mmol/l 1.0–1.8 mmol/l in children	C (5 ml)
Phosphatase, acid	1–5 KA unit	1.77	1–7 iu/l (37°C)	C (5 ml)
alkaline	3–13 KA unit	7.1	20–90 iu/l (37°C) <150 in children	C (5 ml)
Phospholipids	5–10 mg%	0.323	1.6–3.2 mmol/l	C (10 ml)
Potassium	15–20 mg% 3.8–5.0 mEq/l	1	3.8–5.0 mmol/l	H (5 ml)
Protein, total	6.2–8.0 g%	10	62–80 g/l	C (10 ml)
albumin	3.6–4.7 g%	10	36–47 g/l	C (10 ml)
globulin	2.4–3.7 g%	10	24–37 g/l	C (10 ml)
IgA	90–450 mg%	—		C (10 ml)
IgG adult	700–1400 mg%	—		C (10 ml)
IgM	50–205 mg% ♂	—	55–220 ♀	C (10 ml)
IgD	0.3–40 mg%	—		C (10 ml)
Protein bound iodine	4.0–7.5 µg%	78.8	300–600 nmol/l	C (10 ml)
Pyruvate	0.4–0.7 mg%	113.5	45–80 µmol/l	(lab. collects)
Sodium	306–329 mg% 135–148 mEq/l	1	135–148 mmol/l	H (5 ml)
Serotonin	0.1–0.35 µg/ml			(lab. collects)
Sulphate	1–18 mg%	0.31	0.312–0.56 mmol/l	C (5 ml)
Thymol turbidity	0–3 units/ml	—	0–3 units/ml	C (2 ml)
Thyroxine-iodine T$_4$	5.0–12.0 µg%	12.9	69–150 nmol	C (10 ml)
Transaminase, SGOT	0–40 units/ml	0.75	4–18 iu/l	C (5 ml)
SGPT	0–12 units/ml	2.0	<23 iu/l	C (5 ml)
Triglycerides	30–150 mg%	0.0113	0.34–1.7 mmol/l	C (10 ml)
Transferrin	120–200 mg%	0.01	1.2–2.0 g/l	C (10 ml)
TSH			<7.5 m.u./l	
Tyrosine	0.5–2.0 mg%	55.2	27.6–110 µmol/l	C (5 ml)
T$_3$ absolute			0.8–2.5 nmol/l	

T₃ Uptake	95–115%	—	95–115%	C (10 ml)
T₄ free			8.24 pmol/l	
Urea	15–40 mg%	0.166	2.5–6.5 mmol/l	H (5 ml)
Urea nitrogen	10–20 mg%	0.166	1.66–3.3 mmol/l	H (5 ml)
Urate	2–7 mg%	0.06	0.1–0.4 mmol/l	C (10 ml)
Vitamin A	20–50 µg%	0.035	0.7–1.7 µmol/l	H (10 ml)
B₁	1 µg%	33.2	33.2 nmol/l	C (10 ml)
B₂	0.3–1.3 µg%	0.0266	0.008–0.0346 µmol/l	C (10 ml)
B₆	3–8 µg%	0.06	0.18–0.48 µmol/l	C (10 ml)
B₁₂			150–1000 ng/l	C (10 ml)
C	0.5–1.5 mg%	56	28.0–84 µmol/l	(lab. collects)
D	70–300 mg%	0.0256	1.79–7.69 mmol/l	
E	560–1950 µg%	0.0235	13.18–45.9	
Volume, blood	49–75 ml/kg body wt.♂; 56–75 ml/kg body wt.♀ 2500–400 ml/m²			Adult values (Section 8.2 for children)
plasma	31–55 ml/kg body wt.♂; 36–50 ml/kg body wt.♀ 1400–2500 ml/m²			
red cell	18–33 ml/kg body wt.♂; 20–27 ml/kg body wt.♀			
Zinc	1–2 mEq/l	0.5	0.5–1 mmol/l	C (10 ml)
Zinc turbidity	2–6 units			C (5 ml)

5

Normal blood values

5.1.2 Routine haematology

All the samples below are collected in an EDTA (sequestrene) bottle

Haemoglobin (Hb)	men	13.5 – 18.0 g/dl
	women	11.5 – 16.5 g/dl
Red blood cell count (RBC)	men	4.5 – 6.0 X 10^{12}/l
	women	3.5 – 5.0 X 10^{12}/l
White blood cell count (WBC)		4.0 – 11.0 X 10^9/l
Neutrophils	40–75%	2.5 – 7.5 X 10^9/l
Lymphocytes	20–45%	1.5 – 3.5 X 10^9/l
Monocytes	2 – 10%	0.2 – 0.8 X 10^9/l
Eosinophils	1–6%	0.04 – 0.44 X 10^9/l
Basophils	0–1%	0 – 0.1 X 10^9/l
Platelet count		150 – 400 X 10^9/l
Reticulocyte count	0 – 2%	of RBCs
Sedimentation rate (ESR)	men	3 – 5 mm in first hour
	women	4 – 7 mm in first hour
Packed cell volume (PCV)	men	0.40 – 0.55
Haematocrit (HCT)	women	0.36–0.47
Mean corpuscular volume (MCV)		76 – 96 fl (femtolitres)
Mean corpuscular haemoglobin concentration (MCHC)		31 – 35 g/dl
Mean corpuscular haemoglobin (MCH)		27 – 32 pg (picograms)

Haptoglobin binding capacity is usually above 1 g of haemoglobin
per litre of plasma. The lower and upper limits of 'normal' vary
widely depending on the clinical state.

Miscellaneous tests

Serum	
Vitamin B12	150 – 1000 ng/l
Folic acid	3 – 20 μg/l

Sequestrene (EDTA)
    Red cell folate   160 – 640 μg/l
Plasma (heparin tube)
    Iron   14 – 30 μmol/l
    Total iron binding
    capacity (TIBC)   45 – 69 μmol/l

5.2 Management of the bleeding patient

When patients bleed unexpectedly, it is always wise to consult a haematologist. Blood tests are only of real value when the following questions have been answered:

5

1 Why is the patient bleeding now?
2 Has abnormal bleeding occurred before?
3 What drugs are being used or have been taken recently?
4 Is there a family history of abnormal bleeding?
5 Are there abnormal physical signs?
    a Purpura?
    b Palpable nodes, liver or spleen?
    c Evidence of previous haemorrhage into joints or muscles?

5.2.1 Coagulation tests

Platelet count. 150–400 X 10^9/l.

Bleeding time. 2 – 9 minutes.
The result of this test varies depending on the site chosen and the method used.

Coagulation or clotting time. 3–11 minutes.
The result of this test varies depending on the method used. It is only of value for monitoring heparin therapy at bedside.

Management of the bleeding patient

Samples for the following tests are collected in citrate tubes. The figures quoted are only guides to the normal ranges which vary between laboratories.

Prothrombin time (PT). 12–14 seconds.
This test measures deficiency of factors I, II, V, VII, X (extrinsic system).

Prothrombin ratio (PTR). 1.0–1.3 $= \dfrac{PT}{control}$

Prothrombin ratios are now widely standardized by use of the British Comparative Thromboplastin. The therapeutic range for oral anticoagulants is approximately 2.0–3.5. The prothrombin ratio is also useful in the diagnosis of hepatic dysfunction.

Thrombotest. Therapeutic range 5–15%.
This is a commercial variant of the prothrombin ratio and is used to monitor oral anticoagulants in some centres.

Partial thromboplastin time (PTT). 35–45 seconds.
This test measures deficiencies of factors I, II, V, X, VIII, IX, XI, XII (intrinsic system). The most common variant of this test is the Kaolin Cephalin Clotting Time Test (KCCT) which uses Kaolin as an activator and Cephalin as a platelet phospholipid substitute. The normal range given above is wide and varies between laboratories. The test is useful for analysis of hereditary clotting defects, intravascular coagulation and monitoring heparin therapy.

Thrombin clotting time (TCT, TT).

Calcium thrombin clotting time. 10–20 seconds.
Sensitive to hypofibrinogenaemia, heparin and fibrinogen degradation products. The test is used for diagnosis of intravascular coagulation and to monitor heparin therapy.

Reptilase time. 17–20 seconds.
Sensitive to hypofibrinogenaemia and fibrinogen degradation products but normal in the presence of heparin. The test is useful in the diagnosis of intravascular coagulation especially in the presence of heparin.

Fibrinogen. 2–5 g/l.
This is useful in the diagnosis of intravascular coagulation.

Fibrinogen degradation products (FDP). <10 mg/l.
This test is useful in the diagnosis of intravascular coagulation. **NB.** the blood is collected in a tube containing thrombin to which EACA has been added.

5

Euglobulin lysis time. >2 hours.
This measures fibrinolytic activator in the blood and is used in the diagnosis of fibrinolytic status.

5.2.2 Haemostasis tests

The table of screening tests opposite gives a rough guide to diagnosis and management of the bleeding patient.

Please note:

1 It is always worthwhile to discuss the results of tests with a haematologist. The problems of further investigation and treatment are often complex and normal routine test results do not rule out a haemostatic defect in all cases.

2 When serious haemorrhage has taken place, it may be difficult to distinguish a primary haemostatic defect from the secondary effect of bleeding and blood transfusion.

3 Where there is an established or suspected defect of haemostasis intramuscular injection should be avoided.

4 Blood samples from patients and from most therapeutic blood products may carry a hepatitis risk to the clinical and laboratory staff. Special care should be taken in the management of high risk patients.

5

Abnormality	Possible diagnosis	Possible management
Platelets reduced; clotting tests normal	Bone marrow failure, e.g. aplasia, malignancy, vitamin deficiency Consumption of platelets, e.g. ITP, hypersplenism	Specific therapy, e.g. folic acid, withdrawal of causative drugs Corticosteroids Platelet infusions
PTR only abnormal	Exclude presence of oral anticoagulants and liver disease Factor VII deficiency rare	If presence of oral anticoagulants is confirmed then consider FFP, vitamin K and/or factor concentrates*
PTT only abnormal	Probable inherited defect of intrinsic pathway, e.g. haemophilia or Von Willebrand's disease. In the latter, platelet function is defective, with long bleeding time	After confirming with specific factor assays, give specific factor concentrate* or FFP as indicated
PTR, PTT abnormal TCT and platelets normal	Typical of oral anticoagulants, liver disease, vitamin K deficiency. Exclude DIC, and inherited defects of II, V, X, which are rare	Vitamin K, FFP, and/or factor concentrates*
PTR, PTT abnormal TCT normal, platelets reduced	Massive blood transfusion Exclude DIC and liver disease	FFP and platelet concentrates
PTR, PTT, TCT abnormal; reptilase and platelets normal	Typical of heparin therapy (or see below)	Exclude haemostasis failure due to heparin Consider withdrawing heparin or using protamine
All clotting tests abnormal. Platelets normal or reduced; red cells fragmented on film	Typical of severe liver disease or DIC	Avoid factor concentrates if possible* In liver disease use vit. K and FFP. In DIC use FFP, platelet concentrates and heparin, after trying to treat underlying condition†

ITP = idiopathic thrombocytopenic purpura. FFP = fresh frozen plasma. DIC = disseminated intravascular coagulation
*Factor concentrates may be dangerous because of a hepatitis risk and the possibility of exacerbating DIC.
†Antifibrinolytic agents should be confined to those patients who show abnormal proteolytic activity in the absence of DIC. They are generally contraindicated in bleeding from the upper renal tract.

5.3 Normal urinary values

Name	Values in current units (per 24 h)	Conversion factor	Values in SI units (per 24 h)
Adrenaline	10–150 μg	0.00546	0.05–0.85 μmol
Ammonium	0.03–1.0 g	59	17.7–59 mmol
Amylase	8000–32 000 units		
Ascorbic acid	15–50 mg	5.68	85–284 μmol
Amino acid nitrogen	50–300 mg	0.714	4–20 mmol
5-Aminolaevulate	0.1–6 mg	7.63	0.8–46 μmol
Aldosterone	<15 μg	2.87	<43.0 nmol
Calcium	100–300 mg	0.025	2.5–7.5 mmol
Chloride	100–300 mEq	1	100–300 mmol
Cortisol	130–360 μg	0.0028	0.36–0.99 μmol (♂)
			0.19–0.77 μmol (♀)
Creatine	20–150 μg	0.00546	0.05–0.85 μmol
	0–50 mg	7.6	0–380 μmol (adult)
			68 μmol/kg (neonate)
Creatinine	1–2 g	8.85	8.85–17.7 mmol
Creatinine clearance	120 ml/min	—	
Copper	10–50 μg	0.0157	0.2–0.8 μmol
Coproporphyrin	100–200 μg	1.53	150–300 nmol
Folic acid	3.5–23.5 μg	—	
Formiminoglutamate	0–30 mg	5.77	0–170 μmol
Galactose tolerance test	<3 g in urine 5 h post-ingestion of 40 g galactose		
Glomerular filtration rate	105–140 ml/min		
Glucose	0–0.2 g%	55.5	0–11 mmol/l
Hydroxyproline	10–30 mg/g creatinine	0.0076	0.08–0.25 mmol
5-Hydroxyindole acetic acid (5HIAA)	3–14 mg	5.23	15–75 μmol
4-Hydroxy-3-methoxy mandelate (HMMA)	2–7 mg	5.05	10–35 μmol

Iodine 131 excretion	30–70% of administered dose in 24 h		
Iron	0.06–1.0 mg	17.9	1.0–18.0 µmol
17 Ketosteroids	10–30 mg	3.47	34.7–104 µmol
Lead	30–80 µg	0.0048	0.14–0.40 µmol
Magnesium	80–120 mg	0.0411	3.3–5.0 mmol
Mercury	0–100 µg	4.98	0–498 nmol
Nitrogen non-protein	10–20 g	0.0714	0.7–1.43 mmol
Noradrenaline	5–100 µg	5.92	29.6–592 nmol
Normetadrenaline	0–1.0 mg	5.5	0–5.5 nmol
Oestriol (after 30 week pregnancy)	8–40 mg	3.47	30–140 µmol
Oestrogens	4–25 µg ♂	3.47	14–86.7 µmol
	4–100 µg non-pregnant ♀	3.47	14–347 µmol
Osmolality	300–1000 mosmol/kg	1	300–1000 mosmol/kg
Oxalate	20–40 mg	0.0111	0.2–0.4 mmol
17 Oxogenic steroids	10–20 mg	3.47	30–79 µmol
17 Oxosteroids	8–25 mg	3.47	30–85 µmol
Phosphate	0.5–1.5 g	32.3	15–50 mmol
Potassium	30–100 mEq	1	30–100 mmol
Protein (albumin)	0–0.1 g	(A/G ratio 0.65)	
Pregnandiol	0–10 mg	3.12	0–3.1 µmol
pH	4.5–8.0		
Phosphatase, acid	164 KA units (♂)	—	
	217 KA units (♀)	—	
alkaline	<6000 KA units (♂)	—	30 000–10 nmol
	<7500 KA units (♀)	—	
Porphobilinogen	0.2–2 mg	4.42	.1–10 µmol
Pregnantriol	0.1–3.0 mg	2.97	0.3–9.0 µmol
Renal plasma flow	500–800 ml/min	—	

5

Normal urinary values

Name	Values in current units (per 24 h)	Conversion factor	Values in SI units (per 24 h)
Sodium	50–200 mEq	1	50–200 mmol
Specific gravity	1003–1030	–	
Sulphur (as SO_3)	0.7–3.5 g	31	21.7–108.5 mmol
Urea	15–35 g	16.6	249–581 mmol
Urea clearance	60–95 ml/min		
Urate	0.2–0.74 g	5.95	1.2–4.4 mmol
Urobilinogen	0–4 mg	1.68	0–6.7 μmol
Uroporphyrin I and III	0–25 μg	1.20	0–30 nmol
Volume	1–1.8 l	1	1–1.8 l
VMA	1.6 μg/mg of creatinine	–	

5.4 Normal CSF values

CSF is normally clear and colourless with the following characteristics.

	Values in current units	Conversion factor	Values in SI units	Remarks
Pressure	70–150 mmH$_2$O	0.133	9.33–20 kPa	
Volume	120–140 ml	1	120–140	
pH	7.30–7.35	—	50–54 mmol/l	(H$^+$ ion)
Lymphocytes	0–5 mm^3	1	0–5 x 10^6/l	
Specific gravity	1007	1	1007	
Osmolality	306 mosmol/kg	1	306 mosmol/kg	
Calcium	2–3 mEq/l	0.5	1–1.5 mmol/l	
Chloride	120–130 mEq/l	1	120–130 mmol/l	
Glucose	40–100 mg%	0.055	2.2–5.5 mmol/l	1.1 mmol/l less than blood sugar
Magnesium	0.45–4.0 mEq/l	0.8	0.36–3.2 mmol/l	
Phosphate	0.4–0.7 mEq/l	0.326	0.13–0.23 mmol/l	
Potassium	3–4 mEq/l	1	3–4 mmol/l	
Protein	15–40 mg%	10	150–400 mg/l	
globulin	0–2 mg%	10	0–20 mg/l	
Sodium	140 mEq/l	1	140 mmol/l	
Urea	8–40 mg%	0.166	1.33–6.64 mmol/l	

Lange curve
  paretic 5554321000: luetic 1233432100: meningitic 0001233210

5.5 Normal stool values

	Values in current units (per 24 h)	Conversion factor	Values in SI units (per 24 h)	Remarks
Bulk	100–200 g	1	100–200 g	
Dry weight	23–32 g	1	23–32 g	
Water content	65%	1	65%	
Fat total	<5 g	1	<5 g	
Fat as stearic acid	<7 g	3.52	<25 mmol	<25% of dry stool
Nitrogen	1–2 g	71.4	70–140 mmol	
Urobilinogen	30–300 mg	1.68	50–500 μmol	

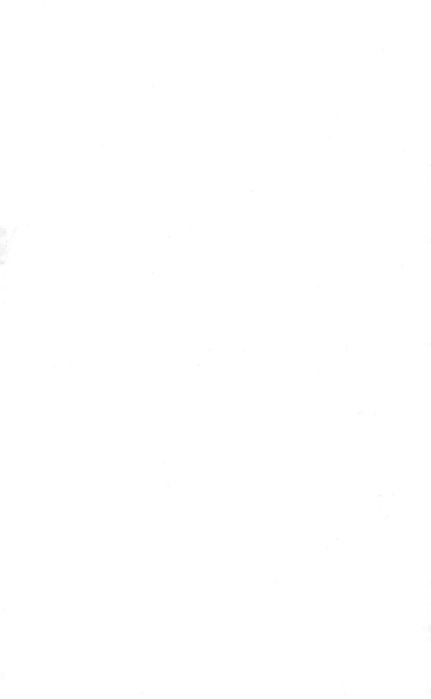

6

6.1 Immediate resuscitation of multiple injuries

Check

1 *Airway and respiration*

Clear foreign material from mouth.

If patient is still clenching teeth, insert Guedel Airway.

If patient is flaccid or respiration inadequate intubate. If this is difficult, maintain on bag and mask.

Check for pneumothorax. Insert chest drain with either underwater seal or, in the field, use Heimlich flutter valve. Rapidly progressive dyspnoea may indicate a tension pneumothorax. Ventilate if necessary.

2 *Circulation*

Set up intravenous infusion for any multiple injuries. Use 16 G or larger plastic cannula. Splint infusion site if over a joint. A patient with 'Multiple Injuries' is unlikely to have lost less than 1000 ml, and may have lost substantially more. Therefore take blood for cross matching and then rapidly infuse Haemaccel 1000 ml minimum, using a pressure infusor.

Set up a CVP line and transfuse to 10 cm H_2O measured from mid axillary line.

3 *Head injury*

Assess level of consciousness using Glasgow Coma Scale. Bear in mind importance of adequate ventilation, proper fluid balance and discriminating use of analgesics in head injury. Look for broken neck.

4 *Catheterize*

Helpful in measuring urine output and detection of urinary tract damage.

5 *Chest X ray*

For detection of pneumo- or haemothorax and correct location of endotracheal tube, chest drains and CVP line.

6

6.2 Cardiac arrest procedure and drug dosages

1 Administer sharp blow to chest (occasional reversal of VF).
2 O_2 – apply facemask and inflate.
3 Intubate and ventilate.
4 Cardiac massage over sternum.
5 Set up intravenous infusion.
6 Give sodium bicarbonate 2–3 mmol/kg over 10–15 minutes.
7 Give calcium (0.1 ml/kg of calcium chloride or 0.2 mg/kg of calcium gluconate). This will counteract the efflux of potassium from the cells due to hypoxia.

8

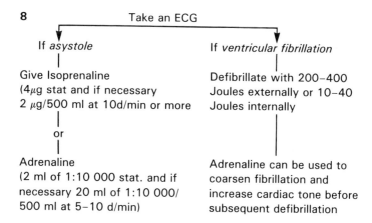

Take an ECG

If *asystole*

Give Isoprenaline
(4μg stat and if necessary
2 μg/500 ml at 10d/min or more

or

Adrenaline
(2 ml of 1:10 000 stat. and if
necessary 20 ml of 1:10 000/
500 ml at 5–10 d/min)

If *ventricular fibrillation*

Defibrillate with 200–400
Joules externally or 10–40
Joules internally

Adrenaline can be used to
coarsen fibrillation and
increase cardiac tone before
subsequent defibrillation

The subsiding metabolic acidosis is treated using sodium bicarbonate 2 mmol/kg over the first hour postarrest. Measure blood gases and electrolytes after 1 hour and 4 hours and repeat bicarbonate if acidosis continues.

Pulmonary oedema is treated with Lasix 80 mg (1 mg/kg)
Cerebral oedema — Some protection may be obtained from mannitol 15–20 g, and Dexamethasone 12 mg
Renal shutdown — Mannitol 0.5–0.75 g/kg or Lasix 1 mg/kg
For treatment of arrythmias see section 4.4

6.3 Diagnosis of brain death

The development of techniques for resuscitation of the cardiovascular system and artificial support of respiration has led inevitably to the problem of some patients being maintained on a mechanical ventilator with a beating heart when the brain is irretrievably dead.

It is now generally agreed that death of the brain·and brain stem function is an indication to withdraw all artificial support. With this in mind the Medical Royal Colleges drew up a joint statement in which they defined a number of conditions that should be satisfied, in order that all forms of support can be withdrawn in the sure knowledge that recovery is no longer possible.

This report was published in full in *British Medical Journal* (1976) **2**, 1187–1188 and the conditions and tests recommended in that report are summarised below.

6

6.3.1 Conditions for considering brain death

All the following should coexist:

1 The patient is deeply comatose.

a Exclude the presence of cerebral depressant drugs, particularly if hypothermia is present or there is a history of drug ingestion.

b Exclude hypothermia, body temperature should be at least 35°C.

c Exclude abnormalities of metabolism or endocrine system. In particular abnormalities of serum electrolytes, acid base balance, blood sugar.

2 The patient is being maintained on a ventilator because spontaneous respiration had previously become inadequate or had ceased altogether. Exclude presence of muscle relaxant drugs or other respiratory depressants.

3 There should be no doubt that the patient's condition is due to irremediable structural brain damage. The diagnosis of a disorder which can lead to brain death should have been fully established.

6.3.2 Tests for confirming brain death

All brain stem reflexes should be absent.

1 The pupils are fixed in diameter and do not respond to sharp changes in the intensity of incident light.

2 There is no corneal reflex.

3 The vestibuloocular reflexes are absent. These are absent when no eye movement occurs during or after the slow injection of 20 ml of ice-cold water into each auditory meatus in turn. Clear access to the tympanic membrane must have been established by direct inspection. This test may be contraindicated by local trauma.

4 No motor responses within the cranial nerve distribution can be elicited by adequate stimulation of any somatic area.

5 There is no gag reflex or reflex response to bronchial stimulation by a suction catheter passed down the trachea.

6 No respiratory movements occur when the patient is disconnected from the mechanical ventilator long enough to ensure that P_{CO_2} rises above 6.7 kPa. Blood gases should be measured and recorded. Patients with pre-existing chronic respiratory disease, may be unresponsive to raised P_{CO_2} and exist on a hypoxic drive to respiration. These cases must be carefully evaluated with blood gas measurements.

6.3.3 Recommended procedure

1 Ventilate with 5% carbon dioxide in oxygen until P_{CO_2} is 5.3–6.0 kPa.

2 Disconnect ventilator and insufflate oxygen into the trachea at 6 litres/min for 5 minutes.

or if blood gas facilities are not available:

1 Ventilate with 100% oxygen for 10 minutes.

2 Ventilate with 5% carbon dioxide in oxygen for 5 minutes.

3 Disconnect from ventilator for 10 minutes while insufflating oxygen at 6 litres/min.

6.3.4 Other considerations

Repetition of testing

It is customary to repeat the tests to ensure that there has been no observer error. The interval between tests varies with the diagnosis and clinical course of the disease. It is common in practice to allow 24 hours to elapse, but this interval might be very much less and no particular time is suggested in the statement.

Integrity of spinal reflexes

Spinal reflexes can persist after irretrievable destruction of brain stem function, and may be present in brain dead patients.

6

Confirmatory investigations

Electroencephalography, cerebral angiography or cerebral blood flow measurements are not necessary to diagnose brain death.

Body temperature

Must be 35° before tests are carried out.

Specialist opinion and status of doctors concerned

Clinicians with wide experience of intensive therapy, acute medicine and accident and emergency should not need specialist advice. If diagnosis is in doubt it is necessary to consult a neurologist or neurosurgeon.

The decision to withdraw support should be made by:
1 The consultant in charge of the case and one other doctor.
2 In the absence of a consultant, his deputy must have been registered 5 years or more and have experience of such cases and one other doctor.

6.3.5 Further developments in the criteria for diagnosis of brain death

Following the publication of the original report referred to above the Conference of Medical Royal Colleges and their Faculties (UK) have published further statements. In 1979[1] an attempt was made to discuss further the implications of death being diagnosed on the basis of brain death as distinct from cessation of heartbeat. In 1980 a code of practice entitled *The Removal of Cadaveric Organs for Transplantation* was published and distributed to all hospital doctors.

In 1981 a further statement[2] was issued in which the following modifications were recommended.

1 The diagnosis of brain death should be made by two medical practitioners, who have expertise in this field. One should be a consultant, the other being a consultant or senior registrar who should assure himself or herself that the pre-conditions have been met before testing is carried out. The length of time required before the pre-conditions can be satisfied varies according to circumstances, and although occasionally it might be less than 24 hours it may extend to several days.

2 The two doctors may carry out the tests separately or together. If the tests confirm brain death they should nevertheless be repeated. It is for the two doctors to decide how long the interval between tests should be but the time should be adequate for the reassurance of all those directly concerned.

3 There may be circumstances in which it is impossible or inappropriate to carry out every one of the tests. The criteria published by the conference give recommended guidelines rather than rigid rules and it is for the doctors at the bedside to decide when the patient is dead.

At the same time a check list was recommended that should be filled in and become part of the hospital record. This has now been done and a new code of practice was published and distributed in 1983 entitled *Cadaveric Organs for Transplantation.* This is now available together with the checklist at all hospitals.

References

1. Conference of Medical Royal Colleges and their Faculties in the United Kingdom. Br Med J, 1979, i, 332. Lancet, 1979, i, 261–2.
2. Br Med J, 1981, 283, 505. Lancet, 1981, ii, 365.

7.1 Hyperglycaemia, with or without acidosis

**Incidence (District General Hospital catchment area 200 000)
20-30 cases per annum**

Mortality: Good centres 10–15%
Average District General Hospital 20–25%
Geriatric patients 50%

Causes of death

1 Delay in diagnosis in primary or secondary health care
2 Delay in treatment
3 Failure to recognize coincidental or precipitating factors (e.g. infection, myocardial infarction, CVA)
4 Inadequate treatment of the diabetes
  (a) not enough fluid
  (b) not enough insulin
  (c) not enough potassium
  (d) failure to correct acidosis
5 Inappropriate treatment: e.g. too much bicarbonate solution
6 No nasogastric tube — aspiration pneumonia

Priorities

1 **Confirm diagnosis at bedside**
  (Primary Health Care or Accident & Emergency)
  (a) blood glucose (dextrostix (Ames) with or without a meter, or glycaeme B.M. sticks (Boehringer))
  (b) Urinary ketones (ketostix, Ames)

2 **Send blood to the laboratory**
Tests for:
  blood glucose
  electrolytes and urea
  full blood picture (for PCV)
  pH (and if possible bicarbonate/Po_2/Pco_2) blood ketones,
  blood for culture

Hyperglycaemia with or without acidosis

7.1.1   Fluid balance

(a) set up i.v. infusion with or without central venous line
(b) start infusion of normal saline ($Na^+ = 155$ mmol/l)
(c) rate of infusion: 1st hour $-$ 2 litres
                     2nd hour $-$ 1 litre
                     3rd hour, etc. $-$ 1 litre
continue this rate of infusion until the patient is clinically
rehydrated or the central venous pressure is normal.

Note: If plasma sodium rises to 155 mmol/l or more then hypotonic
saline should be given. When blood glucose falls to 10 mmol/l or
less, 5% or 10% Dextrose should be given.

7.1.2   Insulin requirements

Start in Primary Health Care or Accident and Emergency

Intramuscular regime (Alberti)

NB Adequate hydration is essential otherwise insulin will not be
absorbed. This regimen is most useful if a high standard of nursing
care is not available.

Regimen:

(1)   At time zero 20 units of intramuscular insulin (soluble, regular
or Actrapid)
(2)   Then every hour 6 u i.m. until the blood glucose falls to
10–15 mmol/l.
(3)   Then 5 units every 2 hours i.m. until the blood glucose
stabilizes at around 10 mmol/l. A three times daily insulin regimen
may then be instituted when the patient starts to feed normally.

Intravenous regimen (Sonksen)

Infusions of insulin i.v. may be given using an infusion pump or by putting the insulin into an infusion of normal saline or Dextrose.
Rate of infusion 4 units per hour until the blood glucose is approximately 10 mmol/l then 1–0.5 units per hour to maintain the blood glucose of 7–10 mmol/l.

7.1.3 Potassium requirements

A failure to correct potassium deficiency is a frequent cause of death in diabetic ketoacidosis.

Replacement regimen

Plasma K+ mmol/l	Dose of KCl:mmol/hr i.v.
Greater than 5	0
4–5	13
Less than 4	26
Less than 3	39

7.1.4 Correction of acidosis

1 Only give bicarbonate solutions if pH is 7.1 or less.
2 Give 8.4% sodium bicarbonate solutions in **50 mmol (50 ml) aliquots** with **13 mmols of potassium added** to each aliquot. This solution should be run in slowly over 20 minutes and after a 10 minute equilibration period the pH should be re-assessed. If the pH is 7.1 or less, 2 should be repeated.

7.1.5 Other considerations

1 Chest X-ray
2 ECG
3 MSU for microscopy and culture
4 Throat swabs
5 Antibiotics
6 Heparinization to prevent DVT and DIC in severely dehydrated unconscious patients.
7 If patient remains oliguric/anuric after rehydration, with a normal central venous pressure and a blood pressure of greater than 100 mm of mercury, treat with i.v. frusemide 120 mg. If this fails to produce a diuresis, treat as acute renal failure
8 Persistent hypotension (BP less than 80 mm of mercury) after 2 hours of adequate hydration with a normal central venous pressure, give blood (2 units)
9 If Po_2 less than 11 kPa (80 mm of mercury) give oxygen therapy

Practical points

1 Blood glucose measured by bedside (Dextrostix – Ames or BM 20–800 strips Boehringer) initially every 30 minutes and then every 2 hours. Laboratory estimation of glucose, potassium, and pH every 2–4 hours
2 Never leave blood glucose estimations to an inexperienced nurse. Inaccurate information is more dangerous than no information
3 In the i.v. regimen Sonksen recommends the addition of albumin, polygeline, purified protein derivative or 2 ml of the patient's blood. (To prevent adhesion of insulin to plastic surfaces)
4 If the intramuscular regimen fails, switch to intravenous regimen (common cause for failure is inadequate rehydration)
5 In the i.v. regimen if blood glucose does not fall, double intravenous dose. Common cause for failure of intravenous regimen is disconnection of the i.v. infusion or pump or an inadvertent switching off of pump

6 Plasma potassium may be high at presentation (i.e greater than 5) because of intracellular acidosis. However, there may be a dramatic fall in the first hour and this must be expected and monitored. The ECG may be helpful but ST flattening and T wave inversion may not be seen until the plasma potassium is less than 2 mmol/l and this is too late!

7 If bicarbonate is given, an extra 13 mmol must be given for every 50 mmol of bicarbonate

8 Gastric atony-dilatation causes
  (a) fluid and electrolyte imbalance, and
  (b) danger of aspiration pneumonia. Therefore **use NG tube**

9 As little as 50 mmol bicarbonate will relieve distressing hyperventilation due to acidosis

10 For every mmol of bicarbonate given, a mmol of sodium is given. There is therefore a danger of hypernatraemia, consequent hyperosmolarity of plasma and therefore intracellular dehydration which might lead to death.

7

7.2   Surgery in diabetes

Cold surgery

7.2.1   Insulin-treated diabetics

1   Admit three days pre-op and stabilize on a thrice daily insulin regimen (Actrapid/Soluble/Regular insulin with a small dose of Monotard/NPH to cover the overnight period). Aim for blood glucose 3–7 mmol/1
2   One day pre-op change to short-acting insulin only (e.g. Actrapid thrice daily)

7.2.2   Suggested PIG regimen

On day of operation set up i.v. infusion ('PIG regimen') of

Potassium as KCL 1 g (13 mmol)
Insulin Actrapid/Soluble/Regular insulin 10 units
Glucose as 10% Dextrose in 500 ml

This 500 ml solution to be run in 4–5 hourly until oral feeding restarts. The insulin dose should be varied as follows

Blood sugar	Insulin dose
Up to 5 mmol/l	5 units
5–9 mmol/l	10–15 units
10–19 mmol/l	15–20 units
Greater than 20 mmol/l	20–25 units/500 ml

The blood glucose, urea and electrolytes to be checked before operation and 2–3 hours after starting infusion. Thereafter the blood sugar should be checked 4 hourly and the urea and electrolytes

8 hourly. Potassium inclusion in the regimen should be varied according to the serum potassium.

When oral feeding begins the infusion should be stopped and the patient should be re-stabilized on a thrice daily Actrapid regimen with the three main meals.

7.2.3 Other considerations

1 If there is evidence of infection, the pre-operative dose will be increased by 20% or more
2 If steroids are administered, the pre-operative dose will also be increased by 20% or more
3 If the patient is fed intravenously, it is important to maintain normoglycaemia (to aid healing and reduce infection) by using an insulin infusion. This is best done with a separate line and an infusion pump
4 When using the PIG or any other infusion regimen it is essential to have a separate i.v. line from that which is being used for other infusions such as blood and saline.

Non-insulin-treated diabetics

If diabetic control is poor, it is better to admit and stabilize on insulin and then use the PIG regimen as above

If control is good (blood glucose 2 hours after a meal 3–7 mmol/l), then on the day of operation the patient should receive no food and no oral hypoglycaemic agent. Long-acting oral hypoglycaemic agent such as Chlorpropamide or Glibenclamide should be stopped 24 hours pre-operatively. Blood glucose should be monitored pre-operatively and during the operation using Dextrostix (Ames) or Glycaemie B.M. strips (Boehringer). If the blood glucose falls below 3 mmol/l then i.v. 5% Dextrose should be given to maintain a blood glucose of between 3–7 mmol/l.

After minor procedures the patient should be re-started on diet with or without a Sulphonylurea with the first normal meal. However, in major procedures it may be necessary to give the patient insulin to maintain the blood glucose at 3–7 mmol/l, as above.

7

8.1 Atoms, molecules and electrolytes

8.1.1 Atomic weight and valency and % human content

	Weight	Valency	% Content by wt in humans
Hydrogen	1	1	10
Helium	4	0	0
Carbon	12	2, 4	18
Nitrogen	14	3, 5	3
Oxygen	16	2	65
Ammonia	17	1	
Fluorine	19	1	0.009
Sodium	23	1	0.109
Magnesium	24	2	0.036
Phosphorus	31	3, 5	1.16
Sulphur	32	2, 4	0.196
Chlorine	35.5	1	0.156
Potassium	39	1	0.2
Calcium	40	2	2.01
Manganese	55	2, 3	0.001
Iron	56	2, 3	0.010
Copper	63.5	2	0.002
Zinc	65	2	0.002
Bromine	80	1	0.002
Iodine	127	1	0.016
Barium	137	2	
Mercury	201	2	
Lead	207	2, 4	
Acetate	60	1	
Bicarbonate	61	1	
Lactate	90	1	
Gluconate	195	1	
Citrate	210	1	

8

8.1.2   Milligram to millmole to milliequivalent conversion equations

$$\text{Milliequivalents/l} = \frac{\text{mg\% x 10 x valency}}{\text{molecular weight}} = \frac{\text{millimole/l x valency}}{}$$

$$\text{Milligrams\%} = \frac{\text{mEq/l x mol. wt}}{10 \text{ x valency}} = \frac{\text{millimoles/l x mol. wt}}{10}$$

$$\text{Millimoles/l} = \frac{10 \text{ x mg\%}}{\text{mol. wt}} = \frac{\text{mEq/l}}{\text{valency}}$$

8.2 Body compartment volumes adults and neonates

	Neonate	Child	Adult
Total body water	75–80% of wt	60–65%	55–60% ♂ 50–55% ♀
Fat	—	20%	11–26% ♂ – ♀
Lean body mass	—	80%	90–74% ♂ – ♀
Blood volume	8–8.5%	7.5%	5.5%–7% (55–72 ml/kg) ♂ – ♀
ECF	45–50%	30–35%	20–25%

8.3 Electrolyte contents of fluid compartments

Electrolyte	ECF (mmol)	ICF (mmol)	Total body amount
Na^+	140	8–10	80 mmol/kg
K^+	3.5	140–150	69 mmol/kg
Ca^{++}	2–2.5	3.5	22.4 g/kg
Mg^{++}	1	15–20	0.47 g/kg
Fe (total)	15–30 μmol	—	75 mg/kg
Cu^{++}	13–24 nmol	—	1.7 mg/kg
Zn^{++}	1 mol	—	28 mg/kg
HCO_3^-	26–30	10	
PO_4^{--}	1.5	50	12.0 g/kg
Cl^-	100	3	50 mmol/kg
SO_4^{--}	0.5	10	
I^-	—	—	0.06 mg/kg

Above figures are adult (66kg) values

8.4 Electrolyte contents of body fluids

Fluid	Na^+ (mmol/l)	K^+ (mmol/l)	HCO_3^- (mmol/l)	Cl^- (mmol/l)	H_2O (ml/24 h)	pH
Sweat	50	10	—	45	500–1000	—
Gastric	60	15	0.15	140	2500	1.5–3.0
Saliva	112	20	10–20	30	500–1500	5–6.5
Bile	140	6	30–50	90	300–1000	5.7–8.6
Pancreatic	130	6	100	60	300–1500	7.7–8.0
Small gut	120	8	20–40	100	1000–3000	6.0–7.0
Diarrhoea	75	30	20–80	—	500+	—
Stools	30	60	20–60	40	100	6.5–8.0
Urine	70	40	—	80	1000–2000	5.5–7.0
CSF	140	4	25	130	100–160	7.32–7.40

8.5 Electrolyte bottle contents (per litre)

Bottle	Strength (%)	pH	Osmolality	Na$^+$	K$^+$	Cl$^-$	HCO$_3^-$	CHO (g/l)	Protein (g/l)	Cal	Misc. (mmol)
				(mmol/l)	Ions						
NaCl (normal)	0.9	5.0	308	150	0	150	0	0	0	0	
NaCl (½ normal)	0.45	5.2	154	77	0	77	0	0	0	0	
NaCl (⅓ normal)	0.30	5.5	114	51	0	51	0	0	0	0	
Dextrose saline {dextrose 4.0 / 1/5 isotonic saline 0.18}		4.5	300	30	0	30	0	40	0	150	
Dextrose saline ½ strength {dextrose 5.0 / ½ isotonic saline 0.45}		4.5	300	77	0	77	0	50	0	188	
Dextrose 5%	5.0	4.0	278	0	0	0	0	50	0	188	
Dextrose 10%	10.0		523	0	0	0	0	100	0	375	
Ringer lactate (Hartmann's)		6.5	280	131	5	112	29 (as lact.)	0	0	9	Mg^{++} 1 / Ca^{++} 1
Ringer lactate ½ strength in 4.5% dextrose		6.0	280	65	2.5	56	14 (as lact.)	45	0	180	
Dextran 40 in 5% dextrose				0	0	0	0	50	0	205	
Dextran 40 in Isotonic saline				144	0	144	0	0	0	0	
Dextran 70 in Isotonic saline				144	0	144	0	0	0	0	
Dextran 70 in 5% dextrose				0	0	0	0	50	0	205	

	conc (%/M)	pH	mOsm/l	Na⁺	K⁺	Cl⁻	HCO₃⁻/lactate	Ca⁺⁺ / Mg⁺⁺	other
NaHCO₃	8.4	8.0	2008	1000	0	0	1000	0	
NaHCO₃	4.2	7.5	1004	500	0	0	500	0	
NaHCO₃	1.4		484	167	0	0	167	0	
Mannitol	10		550					0	
Mannitol	20		1100					0	
Ammonium chloride	⅙M		338	0	0	168	0	0	NH₄ *168
Na lactate	⅙M			167	0	0	167 (as lact.)	0	
Haemaccel	3.5			145	5	145		Ca⁺⁺ 6.25	160
Gelofusine	4		290	154	0.4	125		Ca⁺⁺ 0.4 Mg 0.4	184 ; 45
Plasma/l		<6.0		152	15+	100		Ca⁺⁺ 2.5	
Blood/l				140	15+	103			0
Packed cell/l				10	30+	26			0
Human plasma protein/l	150			150	2	120			39

8

8.6 Drip rates for standard infusion sets

Microdrop. 60 drops/ml = 1 ml/min e.g. Soluset type

1 ml/h	= 1 d/min	= 24 ml/day
5	= 5	= 120
21	= 21	= 500
42	= 42	= 1000
100	= 100	= 2400
126	= 126	= 3000
200	= 200	= 4800

Standard. 20 drops/ml = 1 ml/min e.g. Baxter/Avon type

1 ml/h	= 0.33 d/min	= 24 ml/day
5	= 1.67	= 120
21	= 7	= 500
42	= 14	= 1000
100	= 33	= 2400
125	= 42	= 3000
200	= 67	= 4800

Others. 10 drops/ml e.g. Haemoset type

1 ml/h	= 0.2 d/min	= 24 ml/day
5	= 0.8	= 120
21	= 3.5	= 500
42	= 7	= 1000
100	= 17	= 2400
125	= 21	= 3000
200	= 33	= 4800

By taking the required ml/h or day and reading across, the correct drops per minute for that infusion set can be found.

8.7 Paediatric fluid and electrolyte requirements

8.7.1 Fluid requirement — children (Liverpool) method

First 10 kg body weight — 100 ml/kg/day = 4 ml/kg/h
Next 10 kg body weight — 50 ml/kg/day = 2 ml/kg/h
Additional body weight — 20 ml/kg/day = 0.8 ml/kg/h

e.g. Child of 30 kg needs 1000 + 500 + 200 ml/day
Less fit children post-op. need less
i.e. 70–80 ml/kg/day for first 10 kg body weight
30–40 ml/kg/day for next 10 kg body weight

8.7.2 A paediatric guide

The chart below shows average healthy values ± 15%, so will only give a guide to parameters.

	Age (years)													
	0	$\frac{1}{4}$	$\frac{1}{2}$	$\frac{3}{4}$	1	2	3	4	5	6	7	8	9	10
Weight (kg)	3.5	5.0	7.0	8.5	10	13	15	17	19	21	23	25	28	32
Height (cm)	50	60	65	70	75	86	97	104	110	115	123	131	135	140
Blood volume (litre)	0.2	0.4	0.52	0.65	0.75	0.9	1.05	1.22	1.37	1.52	1.7	1.9	2.06	2.4
Haemoglobin (g)	18	10	11	11.5	12	12.7	13.1	13.3	13.5	13.6	13.7	13.8	13.9	14
Haematocrit (%)	61	30	32	34	36	37	37.6	38.2	38.8	39.5	40	40.5	41	42
Water (ml/kg/day)	130	125	120	115	110	102	95	93	90	86	82	78	76	75
Na and K (mmol/kg/day)	4	3.7	3.3	3.0	2.8	2.5	2	1.98	1.95	1.90	1.85	1.8	1.75	1.7
Calories (kcal/day)	112	111	109	107	105	101	98	97	96	93	90	85	80	75
Urine (ml/day)	280	300	340	370	400	450	500	530	560	640	700	750	800	850
Insensible loss (ml/kg)	31	30	29	28	27.5	27	26.5	26	25	24	23	22	21	20

8.8 Electrolyte, fluid and nutritional requirements

Average minimum daily requirements per kg for adults, children and neonates over 10 kg in weight.

	Adults (per kg)	Children and neonates (per kg)
Water	30–35 ml	100–150 ml
Energy	35–40 kcal (0.15 MJ)	90–125 kcal (0.38–0.5 MJ)
Cal: N_2 ratio	1:200	1:300
Amino acids (nitrogen)	90 mg	330–350 mg
Protein	0.6–0.9 g	1.8 g
Glucose	2–3 g	12–18 g
Fat	2 g	4 g
Na^+	1–1.4 mmol	1–2.5 mmol
K^+	0.7–0.9 mmol	2 mmol
Ca^{++}	0.11 mmol	0.5–1 mmol
Mg^{++}	0.04 mmol	0.15 mmol
Fe^{++}	1 μmol	2 μmol
Mn^{++}	0.6 μmol	1 μmol
Zn^{++}	0.3 μmol	0.6 μmol
Cu^+	0.07 μmol	0.3 μmol
Cl^-	1.3–1.9 mmol	1.8–4.3 mmol
P^{--}	0.15 nmol	0.4–0.8 nmol
F^-	0.7 μmol	3.0 μmol
I^-	0.015 nmol	0.04 nmol
Retinol (Vit. A)	10 μg	0.1 mg
Thiamine (Vit. B_1)	0.025 mg	0.06 mg
Riboflavine (Vit. B_2)	0.03 mg	0.08 mg
Nicotinamide	0.03 mg	0.8 mg
Pyridoxine (Vit. B_6)	0.03 μg	0.1 mg
Folic acid	3 μg	20 μg
Cyanocobalamin (Vit. B_{12})	0.03 μg	0.2 μg
Pantothenic acid	0.2 mg	1 mg
Biotin	5 μg	30 μg
Ascorbic acid (Vit. C)	1.0 mg	3 mg
Ergocalciferol (Vit. D)	0.04 μg	2.5 μg
a-Tocopherol (Vit. E)	1.5 mg	3.0 mg
Phytomenandione (Vit. K)	2 μg	50 μg

8

8.8.1 Basal metabolic rate chart

The following shows basal metabolic rates in energy/m^2 body surface/hour (reproduced from Robertson JD & Reid DD (1952) *Lancet,* **i**, 940).

Age (years)	Males kcal	Males MJ	Females kcal	Females MJ
3	51.1–68.8	0.215–0.288	46.4–62.6	0.194–0.261
5	47.7–65.0	0.198–0.271	44.9–61.1	0.288–0.255
7	43.4–60.7	0.181–0.253	42.1–58.3	0.176–0.243
9	39.6–56.3	0.165–0.235	38.2–54.5	0.159–0.227
11	37.7–52.2	0.157–0.218	35.1–50.6	0.146–0.211
13	36.0–49.3	0.150–0.206	33.2–45.1	0.139–0.188
16	33.7–46.9	0.141–0.196	31.3–40.8	0.131–0.171
19	32.7–45.0	0.137–0.188	29.7–39.3	0.124–0.164
22	32.4–43.1	0.135–0.180	29.2–38.8	0.122–0.162
30	31.4–41.4	0.131–0.173	29.2–38.9	0.122–0.163
40	30.5–40.5	0.127–0.169	27.8–37.5	0.116–0.157
50	28.8–38.8	0.120–0.162	27.1–36.7	0.113–0.153
60	28.1–38.1	0.117–0.159	26.5–36.1	0.111–0.151
70	27.4–37.4	0.114–0.156	25.9–35.5	0.108–0.148

8.9. Parenteral nutrition

8.9.1. Parenteral nutrition bottle contents (per litre)

Bottle	Strength	pH	Osmolality	Na+	K+	Cl−	N2 (g)	CHO (g)	Protein (g)	kcal	Misc. additives (mmol)
Sorbitol	30	6.0	2100	0	0	0	0	300	0	1200	0
Dextrose	10	5.6	523	0	0	0	0	100	0	400	0
Dextrose	20	5.6	1250	0	0	0	0	200	0	800	0
Dextrose	50	5.6	3800	0	0	0	0	500	0	2000	0
Fructose	25		1500	0	0	0	0	250	0	1000	0
Ethanol	5			0	0	0	0	50	0	350	0
Normodex	15	5.2	945	40	20	40	0	150	0	615	Mg 1.5; Lactate 23
Glucoplex	1000		1500	50	30	67	0	250	0	1000	Mg 2.5 PO$_4$ 18, Zn 0.46
Glucoplex	1600		2800	50	30	67	0	400	0	1600	Mg 2.5 PO$_4$ 18, Zn 0.46
Plasma-Lyte M				40	16	40	0	48	0	191	Ca 2.5, Lactate 12, Mg 1.5
Vamin N	9	5.2		50	20	55	9.4	0	60	239	Ca 2.5, Mg 1.5
Vamin glucose	9	7.4		50	20	55	9.4	100	60	650	Mg 1.5, Ca 2.5
Aminoplex	5		1275	35	28	62	6	175	35	1000	Mg 4.5 + Alcohol + Sorbitol
Aminoplex	12	7.4	800	35	30	67	12.4	0	78	316	Mg 2.5
Aminoplex	14	7.4	960	35	30	81	13.4	0	84	340	
Aminofusin	600	0.8		40	30	14	7.6	100	48	626	Mg 5.0 + Sorbitol
Aminofusin	1000			40	30	14	7.6	250	48	1000	Mg 5, Sorbitol + Ethanol
Synthamin	9	6.0		73	60	70	9.3	0	57	236	PO$_4$ 30
Synthamin	14	6.0		73	60	70	14.3	0	90	363	PO$_4$ 30
Synthamin	17	6.0		73	60	70	16.9	0	105	429	PO$_4$ 30
Perifusin	5			40	30	9	5	0	31		Mg 5
Freamine II	12			10	0	0	12.6	0	79		PO$_4$ 10
Intralipid	10	7.0	280	0	0	0	0	0	0	1000	Soya bean
Intralipid	20	7.0	330	0	0	0	0	0	0	2000	Soya bean
Lipiphysan	10			0	0	0	0	0	0	1240	Cotton seed
Lipiphysan	15			0	0	0	0	0	0	1780	Cotton seed

Parenteral nutrition

8.9.2 Calorific values of nutrients

	Calorific value (Cal/g)	Respiratory quotient
Fat	9.0	0.7
Alcohol	7.0	0.66
Protein	4.2	0.8
CHO	4.0	1.0

RQ normally 0.8 (on average diet)

CHO = carbohydrate

8.9.3 Daily nitrogen loss

Calculated in g of N_2 :

1 Urine loss $\quad = $ 24 hour urine urea in mmol x $\dfrac{3.38}{100}$

2 Blood urea correction $= $ increase in blood urea in mmol/l x

$$wt\,(kg) \times \frac{17.35}{1000}$$

3 Proteinuria loss $\quad = $ proteinuria in g/24 h x 0.16

Add **1** to **2** to **3** for total N_2 loss per day

1 g N_2 = 6.25 g protein = 25.3 g of wet muscle
200 cal of CHO needed to utilize 1 g of N_2

8.9.4 Adjusted calcium levels for albumin

Adjusted Ca^+ mmol/l = total $Ca - [0.025 \times Alb] + 1$ to albumin of 40 g/l

8.9.5 Regimens for parenteral nutrition

It is important when planning parenteral nutrition to remember the following:

1 Keep ratio of 200 cal of CHO to 1 g N_2.

2 Add vitamins, e.g. solvito vitalipid multibionta.

3 Add trace elements, e.g. Mg, Mn, Cu, Zn or as addamel.

4 Add phosphate, e.g. $K.H_2PO_4$ or polyfusor phosphate.

5 Add folic acid 10 mg/day.

6 Do not add any drugs to actual feeding line when it is running into patient. Any addition should be added aseptically before.

7 Monitor electrolytes daily, both serum and urine. Monitor urine or blood sugar at least four times a day. Monitor acid base status and LFTs at least weekly.

8

Parenteral nutrition

8.9.6   Suggested regimens

For 66 kg adult with moderate catabolism.

Regimen		ml	Cal	N$_2$ (g)	Additives
1	Glucose 50%	1000	2000	13.4	Add vitamins,
	Glucose 20%	1000	800		trace elements
	Aminoplex 14	1000	380		+ insulin
2	Glucose 20%	1000	800	9.4	Add vitamins,
	Vamin glucose	1000	650		trace elements
	Intralipid 10%	500	1000		+ insulin
3	Glucoplex 1600	1000	1600	12.4	
	Glucoplex 1000	1000	1000		
	Aminoplex 12	1000	316		
4	Aminoplex 5	3000	3000	18	Watch for acidosis add
					vitamins and trace elements

When fat solutions are not used in the regimen add two bottles Intralipid weekly

Suggested 3 litre bag premixed feed

(Plain)		(Intralipid)	
Vamin glucose 10%	1500 ml	Vamin glucose 10%	1500 ml
Dextrose 50%	1000 ml	Dextrose 20%	1000 ml
Dextrose 20%	500 ml	Intralipid 20%	500 ml
Folic acid	6–10 mg	Folic acid	10 mg
Potassium	100 mmol	Potassium	92 mmol
Sodium	90 mmol	Sodium	98 mmol
Phosphate	60 mmol	Phosphate	38 mmol
Solvito	1 vial	Solvito	1 vial
Addamel	1 vial	Addamel	1 vial
Insulin	80–120 units	Vitalipid	1 vial

8.10 Enteral feeds

8.10.1 Nutrient content of enteral feeds (per 2000 ml)

Name	No. packs	Cal	Protein (g)	Fat (g)	CHO (g)	Ca	P	Mg	Na	K	Osmolality	Form	NG tube	Trace elements vitamins	Comments
London Hospital Feed	4 x 500 ml cartons	2270	100	120	174	84	86	14	63	111	369	Liq.	Ryles tube	+ +	High Ca^{++} and lactose. Flexible for patient
Clinifeed 400 vanilla	5 cans	2000	80	72	294	27	39	11	53	62	540	Liq.	Fine bore	+ +	Needs to be diluted
Clinifeed 400 choc	5 cans	2000	80	72	294	27	50	31	53	105	540	Liq.	Ryles tube	+ +	Shake well due to sediment
Clinifeed 500	5 cans	2000	160	58	374	18	48	10	51	94	650	Liq.	Fine bore	+ +	Add CHO to get N_2 ratio 1:200
Clinifeed LLS	5 cans	2000	120	80	368	18	34	5	28	52	590	Liq.	Ryles tube	+ +	
Trisorbin	5 sachets	2000	80	80	238	26	38	15	85	85	200	Powd.	Ryles tube	− +	Needs to be mixed to solution
Isocal	6 cans	2190	73	94	280	34	36	19	49	72	290	Liq.	Fine bore	+ +	Very good for standard
Flexical	1 can	2000	45	68	304	30	32	17	30	64	550	Powd.	Fine bore	+ +	Needs to be mixed up
Vivonex HN	8 sachets	2400	82	2	504	2	29	16	8	4	800	Powd.	Fine bore	+ +	Free amino acids poorly absorbed
Aminutrin	4 sachets	235	57	0	0	0	0	0	0	0	−	Powd.	Ryles tube	− −	Needs to be mixed with Calonutrin with added vitamins and trace elements
Calonutrin	6 sachets	2460	0	0	600	0	0	0	24	2	−	Powd.	Ryles tube	− −	
Complan	500 g from packet	2155	100	80	265	93	96	13	87	107	−	Powd.	Ryles tube	+ +	Mix up with milk or water
Nutraxil	5 bottles	2500	95	85	345	33	50	13	83	80	−	Liq.	Ryles tube	− +	

Minerals (mmol): Ca, P, Mg, Na, K

8

Enteral feeds

8.10.2   Composition of three easily made up feeds

For special requirements see hospital dietician.

1   London Hospital Tube Feed:
      1800 ml milk
      100 g skimmed milk powder
      100 ml Prosparol
      66 g Caloreen
      Vitamins added
Contents. 200 ml; 100 g protein; 120 g fat; 197 g CHO; 2268 cal.

2   57 g Casilan
      1 bottle Hycal
      250 ml Prosparol
      150 ml yoghurt
      6 g NaCl + KCl
      Vitamins and trace elements added to 950 ml H_2O
Contents. 1500 ml; 64 g protein; 125 g fat; 106 g CHO; 2285 cal.
This feed is hyperosmolar and is better suited to continuous infusion

3   1000 ml
      2 eggs
      500 g Caloreen
      2 g NaCl
      3 g KCl
      Vitamins and trace elements added to 1000 ml H_2O
Contents. 200 ml; 55 g protein; 500 g CHO; 2850 cal.

SECTION 9
LUNG FUNCTION

9.1 Ventilatory abbreviations

In order to save time and space, many abbreviations are used in pulmonary and cardiac physiology. They are suitably divided into primary symbols, written in capitals, and secondary symbols, written in capitals or small letters in the inferior position typographically.

Primary symbols

C concentration of gas in blood phase
D diffusing capacity
F fractional concentration in the dry gas phase
P gas pressure, i.e. partial pressure
Q volume of blood
R respiratory exchange ratio
S saturation of haemoglobin with oxygen or carbon dioxide
V gas volume

Secondary symbols

A alveolar gas
a arterial gas
B barometric
c pulmonary capillary blood
D dead space gas
E expired gas
I inspired gas
T tidal gas
v venous blood

A dash above a symbol indicates the mean value, e.g. $\bar{V}$ = mean volume of gas. A dot above a symbol indicates per unit time, e.g. $\dot{V}$ = volume of gas per unit time.

STPD = Standard Temperature and Pressure Dry
BTPS = Body Temperature and Pressure Saturated with water vapour
ATPS = Ambient Temperature and Pressure Saturated with water vapour

Examples

$P_A co_2$ = partial pressure of carbon dioxide in alveolar gas
$\dot{Q}$ = volume of blood per unit time, or cardiac output
$F_I O_2$ = fractional concentration of inspired oxygen
P_B = barometric pressure

9

9.2 Respiratory and ventilatory parameters

These values are for adults, with the neonatal figures where applicable. The recognized abbreviations are also shown.

	Adult (66 kg)		Neonate (3 kg)
Lung weight	80 g		50 g
Number of airways	14×10^6		1.5×10^6
Number of alveoli	296×10^6		24×10^6
Work of quiet breathing	4.9 J/min		
Maximum work of breathing	98 J/min		
Pulmonary capillary blood flow ($\dot{Q}_c$)	5400 ml/min		
Pulmonary capillary blood volume (Q_c)	60 ml		
Pulmonary capillary pressure (P_c)	8 mmHg (1.07) kPa		
Respiratory rate	12–14/min		30–50/min
Dead space (V_D)	150 ml	2.2 ml/kg	6–8 ml
Alveolar ventilation (V_A)	4.2 l/min	2–2.5 l/min/m²	300–400 ml
Tidal volume (V_T)	400–600 ml	7–10 ml/kg	16–18 ml
Minute volume (V_{min})	5000–6000 ml/min	100 ml/kg	600 ml/min
Total lung capacity (TLC)	5000–6500 ml		900 ml
Inspiratory reserve volume (IRV)	3300–3750 ml		
Expiratory reserve volume (ERV)	950–1200 ml		
Functional residual capacity (FRC)	2300–2800 ml		
Residual volume (RV)	1200–1700 ml		
Inspiratory capacity (IC)	3600–4300 ml		
Vital capacity (VC)	4200–4800 ml	52 ml/kg	100 ml
Forced expiratory volume in 1 second (FEV_1)	75% of VC		
Peak expiratory flow rate (PEF)	400 l/min	(710–4½ x age)	See below for more accurate assessment
Peak inspiratory flow rate	300 l/min		
Maximum ventilatory volume (MVV)	120 l/min	$35 \times FEV_1$	
Diffusing capacity of carbon monoxide (DCO)	17–20 ml CO/min/mmHg		
Fractional carbon monoxide uptake	53%		
Total compliance of lung & chest wall	0.1 l/cm H_2O		
Compliance of chest wall	0.2 l/cm H_2O		
Compliance of lung	0.2 l/cm H_2O		
Airways resistance	1.6 cm H_2O/l/s		

All these cardiorespiratory parameters are subject to age and weight variations. These results are given after practice runs.

9.3 Lung volumes and capacities

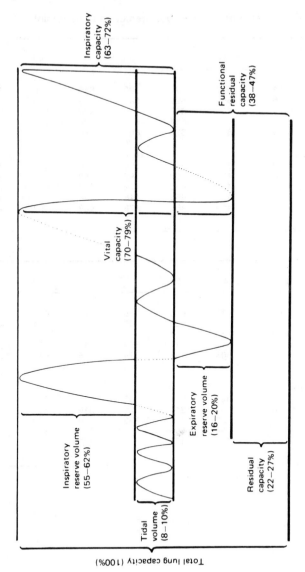

Given as percentage of total lung capacity, an average of 6000 ml for adult, down to 900 ml for 10 kg child.

Inspiratory capacity (63–72%)

Functional residual capacity (38–47%)

Vital capacity (70–79%)

Inspiratory reserve volume (55–62%)

Expiratory reserve volume (16–20%)

Tidal volume (8–10%)

Residual capacity (22–27%)

Total lung capacity (100%)

9.4 Pulmonary function tables

9.4.1 Peak expiratory flow rate prediction table (l/min)

Height			Age (years)					
cm	ft	in	20	25	30	35	40	45
Males								
160	5	3	572	572	560	548	536	524
168	5	6	597	597	584	572	559	547
175	5	9	625	625	612	599	586	573
183	6	0	654	654	640	626	613	599
191	6	3	679	679	665	650	636	622
Females								
145	4	9	377	377	366	356	345	335
152	5	0	403	403	392	382	371	361
160	5	3	433	433	422	412	401	391
168	5	6	459	459	448	438	427	417
175	5	9	489	489	478	468	457	447

Height			Age (years)					
cm	ft	in	50	55	60	65	70	75
Males								
160	5	3	512	500	488	476	464	452
168	5	6	534	522	509	496	484	472
175	5	9	560	547	533	520	507	494
183	6	0	585	572	558	544	530	516
191	6	3	608	593	579	565	551	537
Females								
145	4	9	324	314	303	293	282	272
152	5	0	350	340	329	319	308	298
160	5	3	380	370	359	349	338	328
168	5	6	406	396	385	375	364	354
175	5	9	436	426	415	405	394	384

One standard deviation = 60 l/min

9.4.2   Vitalograph

A good picture of respiratory function can be obtained from this graph. If successive tests are performed, this will give an indication of the progress of the lung disease and its treatment.

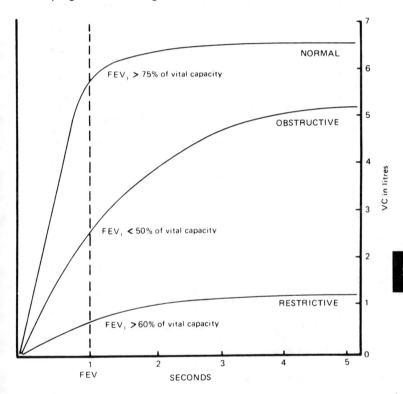

In obstructive lung disease the slope of the graph is depressed
In restrictive lung disease the ultimate vital capacity is reduced

9.4.3   Forced vital capacity prediction table (litres)

Height			Age (years)					
cm	ft	in	20	25	30	35	40	45
Males								
160	5	3	4.17	4.17	4.06	3.95	3.84	3.73
168	5	6	4.53	4.53	4.42	4.31	4.20	4.09
175	5	9	4.95	4.95	4.84	4.73	4.62	4.51
183	6	0	5.37	5.37	5.26	5.15	5.04	4.93
191	6	3	5.73	5.73	5.62	5.51	5.40	5.29
Females								
145	4	9	3.13	3.13	2.98	2.83	2.68	2.53
152	5	0	3.45	3.45	3.30	3.15	3.00	2.85
160	5	3	3.83	3.83	3.68	3.53	3.38	3.23
168	5	6	4.20	4.20	4.05	3.90	3.75	3.60
175	5	9	4.53	4.53	4.38	4.23	4.08	3.93

Height			Age (years)					
cm	ft	in	50	55	60	65	70	75
Males								
160	5	3	3.62	3.51	3.40	3.29	3.18	3.07
168	5	6	3.98	3.87	3.76	3.65	3.54	3.43
175	5	9	4.40	4.29	4.18	4.07	3.96	3.85
183	6	0	4.82	4.71	4.60	4.49	4.38	4.27
191	6	3	5.18	5.07	4.96	4.85	4.74	4.63
Females								
145	4	9	2.38	2.23	2.08	1.93	1.78	1.63
152	5	0	2.70	2.55	2.40	2.25	2.10	1.95
160	5	3	3.08	2.93	2.78	2.63	2.48	2.33
168	5	6	3.45	3.30	3.15	3.00	2.85	2.70
175	5	9	3.78	3.63	3.48	3.33	3.18	3.03

Males: one standard deviation = 0.6 litres

Females: one standard deviation = 0.4 litres

9.4.4 Vital capacity in children

Boys   4– 9 years = (193 x age in years) + 88
      10–12 years = (194 x age in years) + 83
Girls   4–11 years = (191 x age in years) − 62
      12–16 years = (200 x age in years) −121

Reference

Cotes J. E. (1979) *Lung Function.* 4th edn. Blackwell Scientific Publications, Oxford.

9.4.5 Forced expiratory volume prediction table (at 1 second in litres)

Height			Age (years)					
cm	ft	in	20	25	30	35	40	45
Males								
160	5	3	3.61	3.61	3.45	3.30	3.14	2.99
168	5	6	3.86	3.86	3.71	3.55	3.40	3.24
175	5	9	4.15	4.15	4.00	3.84	3.69	3.53
183	6	0	4.44	4.44	4.28	4.13	3.97	3.82
191	6	3	4.69	4.69	4.54	4.38	4.23	4.07
Females								
145	4	9	2.60	2.60	2.45	2.30	2.15	2.00
152	5	0	2.83	2.83	2.68	2.53	2.38	2.23
160	5	3	3.09	3.09	2.94	2.79	2.64	2.49
168	5	6	3.36	3.36	3.21	3.06	2.91	2.76
175	5	9	3.59	3.59	3.44	3.29	3.14	2.99

Height			Age (years)					
cm	ft	in	50	55	60	65	70	75
Males								
160	5	3	2.83	2.68	2.52	2.37	2.21	2.06
168	5	6	3.09	2.93	2.78	2.62	2.47	2.31
175	5	9	3.38	3.22	3.06	2.91	2.75	2.60
183	6	0	3.66	3.51	3.35	3.20	3.04	2.89
191	6	3	3.92	3.76	3.61	3.45	3.30	3.14
Females								
145	4	9	1.85	1.70	1.55	1.40	1.25	1.10
152	5	0	2.08	1.93	1.78	1.63	1.48	1.33
160	5	3	2.34	2.19	2.04	1.89	1.74	1.59
168	5	6	2.61	2.46	2.31	2.16	2.01	1.86
175	5	9	2.84	2.69	2.54	2.39	2.24	2.09

9

Males: one standard deviation = 0.5 litres

Females: one standard deviation = 0.4 litres

9.5 Gases (at P B 760 mmHg or 101.1 kPa)

9.5.1 Normal partial pr sure of gases

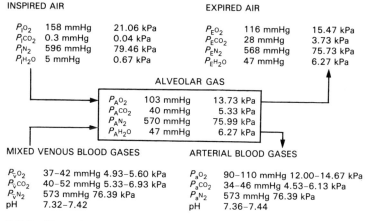

INSPIRED AIR

P_IO_2	158 mmHg	21.06 kPa
P_ICO_2	0.3 mmHg	0.04 kPa
P_IN_2	596 mmHg	79.46 kPa
P_IH_2O	5 mmHg	0.67 kPa

EXPIRED AIR

P_EO_2	116 mmHg	15.47 kPa
P_ECO_2	28 mmHg	3.73 kPa
P_EN_2	568 mmHg	75.73 kPa
P_EH_2O	47 mmHg	6.27 kPa

ALVEOLAR GAS

P_AO_2	103 mmHg	13.73 kPa
P_ACO_2	40 mmHg	5.33 kPa
P_AN_2	570 mmHg	75.99 kPa
P_AH_2O	47 mmHg	6.27 kPa

MIXED VENOUS BLOOD GASES

$P_{\bar{v}}O_2$	37–42 mmHg 4.93–5.60 kPa
$P_{\bar{v}}CO_2$	40–52 mmHg 5.33–6.93 kPa
$P_{\bar{v}}N_2$	573 mmHg 76.39 kPa
pH	7.32–7.42

ARTERIAL BLOOD GASES

P_aO_2	90–110 mmHg 12.00–14.67 kPa
P_aCO_2	34–46 mmHg 4.53–6.13 kPa
P_aN_2	573 mmHg 76.39 kPa
pH	7.36–7.44

9.5.2 Normal content of gases

Inspired: C_IO_2 20.93%   Mixed Venous: $C_{\bar{v}}O_2$ 15%   Arterial: C_aO_2
       C_ICO_2 0.03% $C_{\bar{v}}CO_2$ 52% C_aCO_2

9.5.3 Oxygen availability to tissues

$$\left[\frac{\text{Hb (g\%)} \times 1.34 \times \text{sat. } O_2}{100} + 0.0225 \times P_aO_2 \text{ (kPa)} \right] \times \text{cardiac output (ml)}$$

(1.34 = the amount of O_2 transported per g of Hb
0.0225 × P_aO_2 (kPa) = the amount of O_2 dissolved in plasma)

$$\text{Normally} = \left[\frac{14 \times 1.34 \times 98}{100} + 0.0225 \times 14 \right] \times \frac{5000}{100}$$

$$\cong 950\text{--}1000 \text{ ml/min}$$

The brain cannot extract O_2 below a lower limit of availability of 450 ml/minute.

9.6 Ventilation equations

9.6.1 Alveolar air equation

$$P_AO_2 = P_IO_2 - \frac{P_ACO_2}{RQ} = 100 \text{ mmHg}$$

(RQ depends on diet — normally 0.8)

An easy method of working out shunt and venous dead space equations is shown below.

9.6.2 Dead space equation

$$\frac{V_D}{V_T} = \frac{P_ACO_2 - P_ECO_2}{P_ACO_2} = 0.3$$

P_ACO_2 is calculated from the alveolar air equation (9.6.1) (usually taken as the same as P_aCO_2)

P_ECO_2 is collected and measured by Campbell's modification of the Haldane apparatus.

9.6.3 Percentage venous admixture equation (or shunt equation)

$$\frac{\dot{Q}_S}{\dot{Q}_T} = \frac{C_cO_2 - C_aO_2}{C_cO_2 - C_{\bar{v}}O_2} = 5\% \text{ of cardiac output}$$

$\dot{Q}_T$ = total flow through lungs; $\dot{Q}_S$ = flow through shunt

C_cO_2 is measured from the alveolar-air equation, it is assumed that $C_cO_2 \equiv C_AO_2$.

C_aO_2 Take arterial and venous blood gases and convert to
C_VO_2 percentage content.

9

9.6.4 Alveolar-arterial oxygen difference

$P_AO_2 - P_aO_2 = $ 5–20 mmHg breathing air (0.66–2.66 kPa)
$= $ 10–60 mmHg breathing 100% O_2 (1.3–7.99 kPa)

If the alveolar arterial difference is 120–300 mmHg (15.9–39.9 kPa) when breathing 100% O_2 then the patient needs 40% O_2 added by mask to maintain arterial PO_2. If it is 350 (46.6 kPa) on 100% O_2 then the patient probably has such a large shunt that this cannot be corrected without assisted ventilation.

Alternatively, if the patient has an alveolar arterial difference of 250 (33.3 kPa) when breathing 50% O_2, then ventilation is probably necessary.

9.6.5 PO_2 reduction with age

The older the patient, the lower the normal P_aO_2. The formula below indicates the expected P_aO_2 of patients pre- and post-op.

Pre-op. fit patient $= 104 - \dfrac{age}{4}$ mmHg ($\times$ 0.133 kPa)

Post-op. 24–36 hours $= 94 - \dfrac{age}{2}$ mmHg ($\times$ 0.133 kPa)

9.6.6 Respiratory quotient

Oxygen consumption $= $ 200–250 ml per min
Carbon dioxide production $= $ 150–200 ml per min

Respiratory quotient $= \dfrac{CO_2 \text{ produced}}{O_2 \text{ consumed}} = 0.8$ on a normal diet

See section 8.9.2.

9.7 Virtual shunt lines

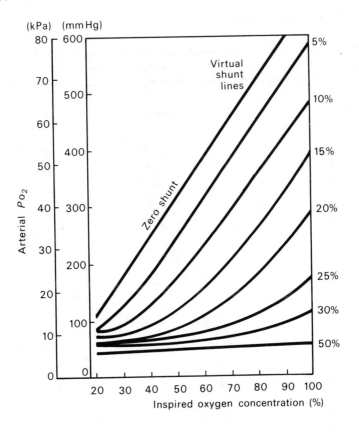

Mean values for arterial P_{O_2} plotted against inspired oxygen concentrations for 15 published studies of anaesthetized patients.

9.8 Basal ventilation requirements

9.8.1 Radford nomogram

Place ruler across patient's weight and breathing frequency. The basal tidal volume can be found. Similarly the frequency of breathing can be estimated from the body weight and tidal volume.

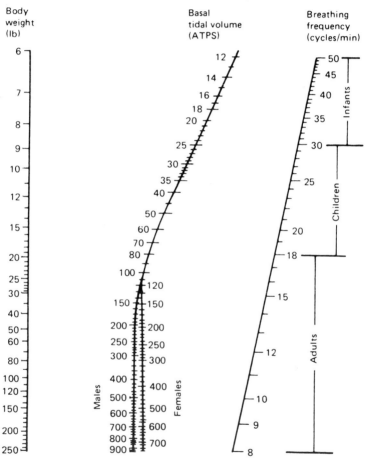

9.8.2   Corrections for Radford nomogram

Correction should be applied as required under the following
conditions

Daily activity	= +	10%
Fever	= +	7.5% for each °C above 38° centrally
Altitude	= +	5% for each 650 m above sea level
Metabolic acidosis		
during anaesthesia	= +	20%

For tracheostomy or intubation the tidal volume (ml) is reduced by
factor of (0.55 x wt (kg))

From **Radford E. P.** (1954) *New Engl. J. Med.* **251,** 877.
Reproduced by courtesy of author and publisher.

9

9.9 Added oxygen to ventilator nomogram

Relating the minute volume, added oxygen and oxygen percentage of resulting mixture. Fix the minute volume and the required O_2 percentage. The O_2 (l/min) to be added is shown in the middle line.

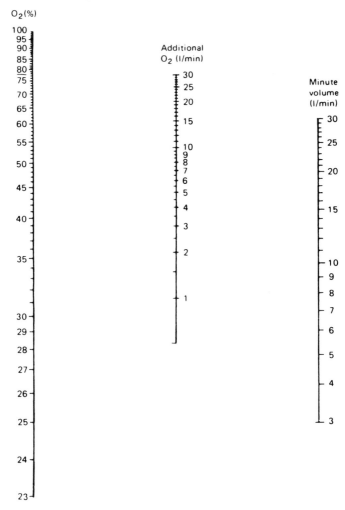

130

9.10 Inspired oxygen to atmospheric pressure nomogram

Relating atmospheric pressure, oxygen percentage and inspired oxygen tension. From the atmospheric pressure and the O_2 concentration percentage, the P_1O_2 can be found.

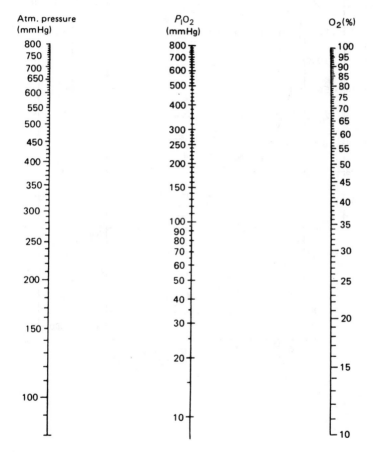

9.9. and 9.10. from **Bird C. G.** (1969) *Anaesthesia* **24,** 38–41. Reproduced by courtesy of author.

9.11 Atmospheric and hydrostatic pressures

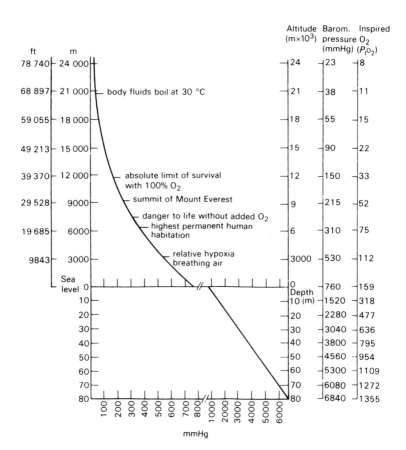

10

10.1 Surface area nomograms

10.1.1 Infants and children
Ventilation, certain drug dosages, basal metabolic rate and lean body mass are more accurately assessed from surface area than from age, weight and height, etc.

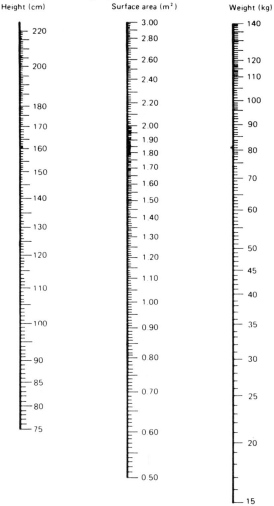

From *Documenta Geigy* (1970) 538 7th edn. CIBA-Geigy, Basle. Reproduced by courtesy of CIBA-Geigy.

10.1.2 Adults

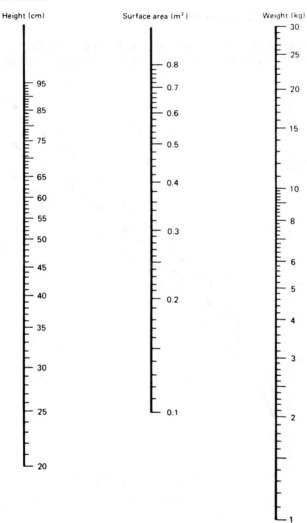

10.2 Percentile graphs

10.2.1 Paediatric age:height

This graph shows height at ages 0–10 years. The 10th, 50th and 90th percentiles shown are each an average of male and female heights.

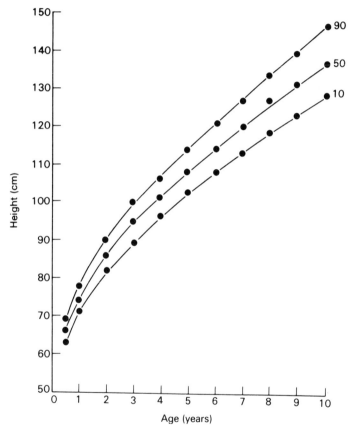

10.2.2 Paediatric age: weight

This graph shows weight at ages 0–10 years. The 10th, 50th and 90th percentiles shown are an average of male and female weights.

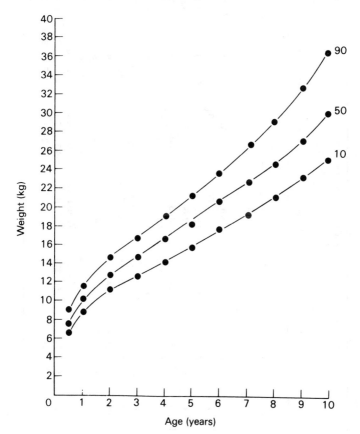

10.2.3 Desirable weights of adults according to height and frame

Desirable weight in kilograms and pounds (in indoor clothing). ages 25 and over

Height without shoes			Small frame		Medium frame		Large frame	
metres	ft	in	kg	lb	kg	lb	kg	lb
Men								
1.550	5	1	50.8−54.4	112−120	53.5−58.5	118−129	57.2−64	126−141
1.575	5	2	52.2−55.8	115−123	54.9−60.3	121−133	58.5−65.3	129−144
1.600	5	3	53.5−57.2	118−126	56.2−61.7	124−136	59.9−67.1	132−148
1.625	5	4	54.9−58.5	121−129	57.6−63	127−139	61.2−68.9	135−152
1.650	5	5	56.2−60.3	124−133	59−64.9	130−143	62.6−70.8	138−156
1.675	5	6	58.1−62.1	128−137	60.8−66.7	134−147	64.4−73	142−161
1.700	5	7	59.9−64	132−141	62.6−68.9	138−152	66.7−75.3	147−166
1.725	5	8	61.7−65.8	136−145	64.4−70.8	142−156	68.5−77.1	151−170
1.750	5	9	63.5−68	140−150	66.2−72.6	146−160	70.3−78.9	155−174
1.775	5	10	65.3−69.9	144−154	68−74.8	150−165	72.1−81.2	159−179
1.800	5	11	67.1−71.7	148−158	69.9−77.1	154−170	74.4−83.5	164−184
1.825	6	0	68.9−73.5	152−162	71.7−79.4	158−175	76.2−85.7	168−189
1.850	6	1	70.8−75.7	156−167	73.5−81.6	162−180	78.5−88	173−194
1.875	6	2	72.6−77.6	160−171	75.7−83.5	167−185	80.7−90.3	178−199
1.900	6	3	74.4−79.4	164−175	78.1−86.2	172−190	82.7−92.5	182−204

Women

			41.7-44.5	92-98	43.5-48.5	96-107	47.2-54	104-119
1.425	4	8	41.7-44.5	92-98	43.5-48.5	96-107	47.2-54	104-119
1.450	4	9	42.6-45.8	94-101	44.5-49.9	98-110	48.1-55.3	106-122
1.475	4	10	43.5-47.2	96-104	45.8-51.3	101-113	49.4-56.7	109-125
1.500	4	11	44.9-48.5	99-107	47.2-52.6	104-116	50.8-58.1	112-128
1.525	5	0	46.3-49.9	102-110	48.5-54	107-119	52.2-59.4	115-131
1.550	5	1	47.6-51.3	105-113	49.9-55.3	110-122	53.5-60.8	118-134
1.575	5	2	49-52.6	108-116	51.3-57.2	113-126	54.9-62.6	121-138
1.600	5	3	50.3-54	111-119	52.6-59	116-130	56.7-64.4	125-142
1.625	5	4	51.7-55.8	114-123	54.4-61.2	120-135	58.5-66.2	129-146
1.650	5	5	53.5-57.6	118-127	56.2-63	124-139	60.3-68	133-150
1.675	5	6	55.3-59.4	122-131	58.1-64.9	128-143	62.1-69.9	137-154
1.700	5	7	57.2-61.2	126-135	59.9-66.7	132-147	64-71.7	141-158
1.725	5	8	59-63.5	130-140	61.7-68.5	136-151	65.8-73.9	145-163
1.750	5	9	60.8-65.3	134-144	63.5-70.3	140-155	67.6-76.2	149-168
1.775	5	10	62.6-67.1	138-148	65.3-72.1	144-159	69.4-79	153-174

Based on weights of insured persons in the United States associated with lowest mortality (*Statist bull Metrop Life Insur Co*, 40, Nov–Dec 1959).

10

10.3 General drugs

10.3.1 Introduction — Pharmacology: Drugs and Doses

The drugs detailed in this section are some of those used most often in hospital practice. Antibiotics and those drugs peculiar to anaesthesia are not included here but are to be found in the sections devoted to those subjects. Drugs used for the cardiovascular system are repeated in the cardiac section.
There are three columns.
1 The non-proprietary name of the drug. A list of proprietary names and their non-proprietary equivalents are to be found in the next section
2 The usual dose for an average-sized adult, including frequency of administration and possible routes. There is a key to abbreviations below. In many cases the initial dose of a drug is increased after a short period to evaluate the clinical effect and these are indicated by the suffix 'Initially'
3 The paediatric dose. In some instances the drug is specifically not recommended for children and this is indicated. In others, there is no mention of a paediatric dose or it is clearly irrelevant and these have been left blank. A general guide to dosage in paediatrics is given in the table below.
Abbreviations
mg = milligram, kg = kilogram, g = gram, ml = millilitres, 4 h = Given at 4-hourly intervals, b.d. = Twice a day, t.d.s = Three times a day, q.d.s. = Four times a day, DD = Divided doses — this is used when the dose given is for a full 24-hour period.
o = oral; i.m. = intramuscular; s.c. = subcutaneous; i.v. = intravenous; B = bolus; I = Infusion; rect. = rectal suppository.

A comprehensive guide to prescribing both in general and in particular situations can be found in the *British National Formulary,* which is published by the British Medical Association and The Pharmaceutical Society of Great Britain and is frequently updated.

If any doubt exists about the dose of a drug, particularly in children, it is advisable to check with the manufacturer's data sheet, your pharmacy, or a paediatrician.

10.3.2 Solution strength conversion table

This is used for drugs and vapours, i.e. 1% solution contains 1 g of substance in 100 ml of solution.

Ratio	Percentage in solution	Concentration (mg/ml)
1:400 000	0.00025	0.0025
1:200 000	0.002	0.02
1:100 000	0.001	0.01
1: 10 000	0.01	0.1
1: 5 000	0.02	0.2
1: 4 000	0.025	0.25
1: 2 000	0.05	0.5
1: 1 000	0.1	1.0
1: 500	0.2	2.0
1: 400	0.25	2.5
1: 100	1.0	10

10.3.3 Paediatric prescribing regimen

Age	Average wt (kg)	Proportion of adult dose (%)
2 months	3.2	10
4 months	6.5	15
1 year	10	25
5 years	18	33
7 years	23	50
12 years	37	75
15 years	55	85
Adult	66	100

10

10.3.4 General drug list

Drug	Adult dose	Paediatric dose
Acebutolol	200 mg b.d. o. initially 5–25 mg i.v. slowly	
Acepifylline	500 mg–1 g t.d.s. o. 500 mg–1 g i.m. i.v.	*Syrup:* 125 mg/5 ml 0–1 yr:2.5 ml (62.5 mg) t.d.s. o. 1–5 yr: 5 ml (125 mg) t.d.s. o. 6–12 yr: 10 ml (250 mg) t.d.s. o. *Rect:* 1–5 yr–200 mg/day 6–12 yr–300 g/day
Acetazolamide	250 mg 6 h o., i.m., i.v.	Infant: 125 mg/day Child: 125–750 mg/day DD o.
ACTH	See corticotrophin	
Adrenaline 1/1000	0.5 mg = 0.5 ml s.c. 1 mg in 100 ml = 10 μg/ml by i.v. infusion	
Allopurinol	100–200 mg/day o. initially then 200–600 mg/day o.	10–20 mg/kg/day o.
Amiloride	5–20 mg/day o.	
Aminocaproic acid	3–6 g 4–6 h o.	100 mg/kg/dose 4–6 h o.
Aminophylline	100–300 mg o. 360 mg b.d. rect. 250 mg i.v. slowly Infusion: 250 mg in 500 ml in 6 h	*Age* *Oral* *Rectal* 0–1 yr 10–25 mg 12.5–25 mg b.d. 1–5 yr 25–50 mg 50–100 mg b.d. 6–12 yr 50–100 mg 100–200 mg b.d.
Amiodarone	200 mg t.d.s. o. 5 mg/kg i.v. Infusion over 30 min in 250 ml 5% dextrose 150 mg i.v. slowly	
Amitryptiline	25 mg t.d.s. o. Initially 10–20 mg q.d.s. i.m., i.v.	Enuresis only
Amylobarbitone	200 mg o. Up to 500 mg i.m. Up to 1 gm i.v.	
Ancrod	Initial dose: 2–3 mg/kg in N Saline 50–500 ml in 8 h infusion. Maintain: 2 units/kg in 25 ml i.v. bolus slowly 12 h Lab control	
Aprotinin	500 000 KI units stat. 200 000 KI units 4 hr i.v. Infusion	As adult in proportion to body weight

Drug	Adult dose	Paediatric dose
Aspirin	600 mg 4 h o.	1–2 yr: 75–150 mg 6 h
	300 mg/day for	3–5 yr: 225–300 mg 8h
	anticoagulation	6–12 yr: 300–400 mg 6 h
Atenolol	50–100 mg daily o.	
	2.5 mg i.v. slowly (max. 10 mg	
	in 20 min)	
	0.15 mg/kg i.v. over 20 min. 12 h	
Atropine	0.3–1 mg i.m. i.v.	0.02 mg/kg
	Also see anaesthetic section	
Azathioprine	1–4 mg/kg/day o.	As adult
	1–2.5 mg/kg i.v. I slowly	
Bamethan	25 mg q.d.s. o.	
Bendrofluazide	2.5–10 mg daily o.	
Betamethasone	0.5–5 mg/day o.	1/4–1/2 adult dose o.
	4–20 mg 6 h i.m., i.v.	0–1 yr: 1 mg i.v.
		1–5 yr: 2 mg i.v.
		6–12 yr: 3 mg i.v.
Bethanidine	10 mg t.d.s. o. Initially	
Benztropine	1–2 mg/day o. Initially	
	1–2 mg i.v.	
Bretylium	5 mg/kg i.m. Repeat 6–8 h	
Bromhexine	8–16 mg q.d.s. o.	Elixir: 4 mg in 5 ml
	8–24 mg/day DD. i.m., i.v.–B.I.	Under 5 yr: 5 ml b.d.
		5–10 yr: 5 ml q.d.s.
		Not by injection
Bumetanide	1 mg daily o.	
	1–2 mg i.m., i.v.	
	2–5 mg by i.v. infusion.	
Buprenorphine	0.2–0.4 mg 6–8 h subling	Not in children
	0.3–0.6 mg 6–8 h i.m.	
Busulphan	0.06 mg/kg/day (max. 4 mg) o.	
	Maintain: 0.5–2 mg/day	
Calcium chloride	2.5–5 mmol i.v.	
Calcium gluconate	Calcium deficiency −	See manufacturers' literature
Captopril	25 mg t.d.s. o. Initially	
Carbamazepine	100–200 mg b.d., t.d.s. o.	10–20 mg/kg/day o. DD.
	Initially	
Carbenoxolone	100 mg t.d.s. o. Initially	
Carbimazole	10 mg t.d.s. o. Initially	>7 yr: 5 mg t.d.s. o.
Chloral hydrate	1–2 g o.	30–50 mg/kg o. (max. 1 g)
Chlordiazepoxide	10 mg t.d.s. o.	5–20 mg/day DD o.
	(Higher dose possible)	
	50–100 mg i.m.	

10

General drugs

Drug	Adult dose	Paediatric dose
Chlormethiazole	Sedation: 1 capsule = 192 mg 2 capsules o. noct. Higher dose in alcohol withdrawal. Infusion i.v.: 8 mg/ml, 1 ml/min *CAUTION: Overdose =* *Anaesthesia*	
Chlormezanone	200 mg t.d.s. o. 400 mg o. noct.	Not in children
Chlorothiazide	500 mg–2 g daily o.	
Chlorpheniramine	4 mg t.d.s. o. 10–20 mg s.c., i.m., i.v. (max. 40 mg/24 h)	Syrup: 4 mg in 10 ml 0–1 yr: 2.5 ml b.d. o. 1–5 yr: 2.5–5 ml t.d.s o.
Chlorpromazine	25 mg t.d.s. o. Initially 25–50 mg 6–8 h i.m. 5–10 mg i.v.	Under 5 yr: 5–10 mg o., i.m. Over 5 yr:1/3–1/2 adult dose t.d.s. o. i.m.
Chlorpropamide	250–500 mg daily o. (100–125 mg in older patients)	
Chlorthalidone	50–100 mg daily o.	Up to 10 kg: 5 mg/kg alt. die o. Up to 5 yr: 50 mg alt. die o. Over 5 yr: 50–100 mg alt. die o.
Choline theophyllinate	100–400 mg q.d.s. o.	Syrup: 62.5 mg/5 ml 3–6 yr: 5–10 ml t.d.s. o. Over 6 yr: 100 mg t.d.s. o. (Tabs).
Chymotrypsin	20 mg b.d. o. 3 days Maintain: 10 mg b.d. o.	
Cimetidine	200 mg t.d.s., 400 mg nocte o. 200 mg 4–6 h i.m., i.v.	20–40 mg/kg/day DD o., i.v.
Clobazam	10 mg t.d.s. o.	Over 3 yr: 1/2 adult dose
Clofibrate	Over 65 kg: 500 mg q.d.s. o. Under 65 kg: 500 mg t.d.s. o.	
Clomipramine	10 mg/day o. Initially 25 mg 6 times/day i.m. 25–50 mg i.v. infusion over 2 h	
Clonazepam	1 mg/day o. Initially 1 mg i.v., – Slow B, I.	Initially: Infants: 0.25 mg/day o. Child: 0.5 mg/day o. 0.5 mg i.v. slowly.
Clonidine	0.05–0.1 mg t.d.s. o. Initially 0.15–0.3 mg i.v. slowly	
Codeine phosphate	10–60 mg 4 h o. 30 mg 4–6 h i.m.	3 mg/kg/day DD o.
Corticotrophin (ACTH)	40 i.u. daily s.c., i.m. initially Reduce dose to response	See manufacturers' literature
Cortisone acetate	Variable dose, usually 25–100 mg daily DD. o., i.m., i.v.	

Drug	Adult dose	Paediatric dose
Cyanocobalamin	1 mg .10 doses at 2 day intervals Then 1 mg/month i.m.	As adult initially then depends on response
Cyclandelate	400 mg t.d.s. o.	Not in children
Cyclizine	50 mg t.d.s. o., i.m., i.v.	1–10 yr: 25 mg t.d.s. o. Not by injection
Cyclopenthiazide	0.25–0.5 mg daily o.	
Dantrolene	25 mg daily o. Initially Hyperpyrexia: 1 mg/kg i.v. Repeat up to 10 mg/kg max.	
Debrisoquine	10–20 mg daily or b.d. o.	Not in children
Desferrioxamine	Iron poisoning: 5–10 g in 50–100 ml water o. 1–2 g 3–12 h i.m. Infusion i.v.: 15 mg/kg/h. max. — 80 mg/kg/24 h	As in adult
Dexamethasone	0.5–2 g daily o. 0.5–20 mg daily DD i.m., i.v. High doses see manufacturers' literature	Reduce dose in proportion to weight
Dextromoramide	5 mg o., s.c., i.m. Initially Increase to max: 20 mg/dose 10 mg rect.	0.08 mg/kg but not recommended
Dextropropoxyphene	65 mg t.d.s., q.d.s. o. Usually used as compound preparation with paracetamol e.g. Distalgesic Tab 2 6 h o.	Not in children.
Diamorphine	5 mg o., i.m., i.v. Extradural: 2–5 mg in 10 ml of N Saline.	
Diazepam	2.5–10 mg o., i.m., i.v.	0.1 mg/kg
Diazoxide	300 mg i.v. rapidly	5 mg/kg i.v.
Dichloralphenazone	2–3, 650 mg tabs, nocte o.	Elixir: 225 mg in 5 ml Up to 1 yr: 2.5–5 ml 1–5 yr: 5–10 ml 6–12 yr: 10–20 ml
Diclofenac	75 mg b.d., o., i.m. Not i.v.	Not in children
Dicyclomine	10–20 mg t.d.s. o.	Syrup: 10 mg in 5 ml Up to 6 months: 5 mg t.d.s. o. 6 months–2 yr: 5–10 mg t.d.s. o. 2–12 yr: 10–20 mg t.d.s. o.

10

145

General drugs

Drug	Adult dose	Paediatric dose
Diflunisal	500 mg b.d. o.	Not in children
Digoxin	0.25–0.5 mg daily o., i.m. Load dose: 0.5–1 mg i.m., i.v. repeat after 4 h	0.01–0.02 mg/kg repeat in 6 h then daily. All routes
Dihydrocodeine	30 mg 4–6 h o. 50 mg 4–6 h i.m.	Over 4 years: 0.5–1 mg/kg 4–6 h o.
Dimenhydrinate	50–100 mg t.d.s. o.	1–6 yr: 12.5–25 mg t.d.s. o. 6–12 yr: 25–50 mg t.d.s. o.
Diphenhydramine	25 mg t.d.s. o. 50 mg nocte	6–12 yr: 25–50 mg t.d.s. o.
Diphenoxylate	1 dose 4 tabs then 2 tabs 6 h o.	1–3 yr: 1 tab b.d. 4–8 yr: 1 tab t.d.s. 9–12 yr: 1 tab q.d.s. 13–16 yr: 2 tab t.d.s.
Dipipanone + cyclizine	1 tab 6 h o.	Not in children
Diprophylline	400 mg 6 h o. 400 mg b.d. rect. 500 mg t.d.s. i.m. 500 mg i.v. slowly	Syrup: 100 mg in 5 ml Up to 1 yr: 0.5–1.5 ml 6 h 1–2 yr: 2 ml 6 h 3–5 yr: 3 ml 6 h 6–12 yr: 5 ml 6 h
Dipyridamole	100–200 mg t.d.s. o.	5 mg/kg/day DD
Disopyramide	100 mg 6 h o. 2 mg/kg i.v. slowly. Max 150 mg Infusion: 0.4 mg/kg/h Max 800 mg/24 h	
Distigmine	5 mg daily o. Increase to max. 20 mg/day 0.5 mg i.m.	Up to 10 mg daily o. depending on age
Dobutamine	Infusion: 50 mg in 100 ml rate depends on effect	
Dopamine	Infusion: 200 mg in 100 ml rate depends on effect usually 5–10 μg/kg/min	
Doxapram	Infusion: 2 mg/ml 0.5–4 mg/min	
Edrophonium	2 mg i.v. initially. 1 mg increments up to 10 mg	Up to 35 kg: 1 mg i.v., 2 mg i.m. Over 35 kg: 2 mg i.v., 5 mg i.m.
Ephedrine	15–60 mg t.d.s. o. Up to 10 mg i.v. 10–30 mg i.m.	Up to 1 yr: 7.5 mg t.d.s. o. 1–5 yr: 15 mg t.d.s. o. 6–12 yr: 30 mg t.d.s. o.

146

Drug	Adult dose	Paediatric dose
Ergometrine	0.5–1 mg o. 0.25–0.5 mg i.m., i.v.	
Ergotamine	1–2 mg o. Repeat ½ hourly up to total of 6 mg/migraine attack 1 mg i.v., i.m.	
Ethacrynic acid	50 mg daily o. i.v. Initially	Over 2 yr: 25 mg daily o. Not parenteral
Ethamivan	50–100 mg i.v. Up to max 250 mg	Oral soln: 12 drops = 25 mg Lingual absn. Infant: 6 drops Child: 12 drops
Ethamsylate	500 mg q.d.s. o., i.m., i.v. 1 g i.m., i.v. stat	Infant: 12.5 mg/kg 6 h i.m., i.v. Child: 250 mg 6 h o., i.v. 500–750 mg i.m., i.v. stat.
Ethosuximide	500 mg daily o. Initially	Under 6 yr: 250 mg daily o.
Fenbufen	600 mg daily o.	Not in children
Fenoprofen	200 mg q.d.s. o.	Not in children
Flavoxate	200 mg t.d.s. o.	Not in children
Fludrocortisone	Replacement: 0.1–0.3 mg/day o. Hyperplasia: 1–2 mg/day o.	Dose adjusted to weight, age and clinical condition
Flunitrazepam	0.5–1 mg nocte o.	Not in children
Fluphenazine	6.25–12.5 mg i.m. initially	Not in children
Flurazepam	15–30 mg nocte o.	
Folic acid	10–20 mg daily o. 5 mg daily i.v.	5–15 mg daily o.
Folinate calcium	15 mg daily o. 3 mg daily i.v. Increase dose with methotrexate-see manufacturers' literature	0.25 mg/kg/day o.
Frusemide	20–80 mg o., i.m., i.v. High dose (250–500 mg). See data sheet	1–3 mg/kg o. 0.5–1.5 mg/kg i.m., i.v.
Furosemide	See frusemide	
Glibenclamide	5 mg daily o. Initially max 15 mg	
Glucagon	0.5–1 unit s.c., i.m., i.v.	As adult

10

147

General drugs

Drug	Adult dose	Paediatric dose
Glutethimide	250–500 mg nocte o.	1–6 yr: 125 mg ò. Over 6 yr: 250 mg o.
Glyceryl trinitrate	GTN-1 tab sub ling. p.r.n. Sustac: 2.5 mg t.d.s. initially Nitrolingual: metered spray o. Percutol: 1–2 in percut. 4 h Tridil: See cardiac section	
Glycopyrrolate	0.2–0.4 mg i.m., i.v. 1–4 mg b.d. oral.	0.004–0.008 mg/kg i.m., i.v, Max: 0.2 mg
Guanethidine	20 mg daily o. 2–10 mg i.m.	
Haloperidol	0.5–5 mg b.d. o. 10–20 mg i.m.	0.05 mg/kg/day o. Not parenteral
Heparin	Load: 5000 units i.v. 10 000 units 6 h by infusion or i.v. injection. Thrombosis prophylaxis: 5000 units s.c. 12 h	
Hyaluronidase	1500 units s.c., i.m.	
Hydralazine	25 mg b.d., t.d.s. o.	
Hydrochlorothiazide	20–40 mg i.v. slowly	
Hydrocortisone	20–30 mg daily o. 100 mg 6 h i.m. for post- operative steriod cover 100–500 mg 6 h i.v.	Up to 1 yr: 25 mg 1–5 yr: 50 mg 6–12 yr: 100 mg or 5–50 mg/kg/day
Hydroxyzine	25–100 mg t.d.s. o.	Up to 6 yr: 30–50 mg/day DD o. Over 6 yr: 50–100 mg/day DD o.
Hyoscine	0.3–0.6 mg s.c. o. 0.4 mg i.m.	0.008 mg/kg i.m. 3–5 yr: 0.075–0.1 mg o. 6–12 yr: 0.1–0.3 mg o.
Imipramine	25 mg b.d. o. Initially	Enuresis only.
Indoramin	25 mg b.d. o. Initially	
Inositol	1 g t.d.s. o.	
Insulin	See section on diabetes	
Ipratroprium	Metered inhaler Ventilator nebuliser: 0.1–0.5 mg q.d.s.	Ventilator nebuliser: Over 3 yr: 0.1–0.5 mg t.d.s.
Iproniazid	100–150 mg daily o. Then reduce to 25–50 mg/day	Not in children

Drug	Adult dose	Paediatric dose
Isocarboxazid	10–30 mg daily o.	Not in children
Isoprenaline	Sustained release tab: 30 mg 8 h o. Initially Infusion i.v.: 1 mg in 100 ml or higher conc. Stat. i.v. dose: 10–20 μg	
Isosorbide	5–10 mg sub ling. 10–30 mg q.d.s. o. Infusion: 2–10 mg hourly i.v.	Not in children
Labetalol	100–200 mg b.d. o. 10–20 mg i.v. repeat depending on effect. Infusion: 1 mg/ml Rate depends on effect.	
Lactulose	Hepatic encephalopathy: 30–50 ml syrup t.d.s.	
Lanatoside C	Load dose: 0.8–1.6 mg i.m., i.v., over 24 h. 0.25–1.5 mg/day o.	0.02–0.04 mg/kg i.v. then 0.01–0.03 mg/kg/day 3DD o.
Levallorphan	0.5–1 mg i.v.	0.05–0.25 mg i.v.
Levodopa	250 mg–1 g daily 5DD initially	
Levorphanol	1.5–4.5 mg b.d. o. 2–4 mg s.c., i.m. 1–2 mg i.v.	Not in children
Lignocaine	100 mg i.v. stat. Infusion: 1–2 mg/min i.v. See also anaesthetic section	
Lithium	0.25–2 g daily o. DD	—
Loperamide	2 tabs initially. Then 1 tab after loose stool Max: 8 tabs/day	Syrup: 1 mg/5 ml 4–8 yr: 5 ml q.d.s. o. 9–12 yr: 10 ml q.d.s. o.
Lorazepam	1–4 mg o. 0.025–0.05 mg/kg i.m., i.v.	Not in children
Lormetazepam	0.5–1 mg nocte o.	Not in children
Mecamylamine	2.5 mg b.d. o. Initially	—
Medazepam	5 mg b.d., t.d.s. o. 10–15 mg o. nocte	1–1.5 mg/kg/day o.

10

General drugs

Drug	Adult dose	Paediatric dose
Medigoxin	Load: 0.2 mg b.d. o., i.v. – 3 days Maintain: 0.1 mg b.d. daily	0.01 mg/kg 6 h 2–4 doses 0.01 mg/kg/day
Mefanamic acid	500 mg t.d.s. o.	Suspension: 50 mg/5 ml Over 6 months: 25 mg/kg/day DD
Menadiol	10 mg daily o. 10 mg i.m.	5 mg daily o.
Meprobamate	400 mg t.d.s. o.	
Meptazinol	75–100 mg 2–4 h i.m. 50–100 mg 2–4 h i.v.	Not in children
Mepyramine	100 mg t.d.s. o. Initially	Up to 3 yr: 12.5–25 mg t.d.s. o. 3–7 yr: 25–50 mg t.d.s. 7–14 yr: 25–75 mg t.d.s.
Metaraminol	5 mg i.m., 1 mg i.v.	
Metformin	500 mg 8 h o.	
Methadone	5–10 mg o., s.c., i.m., i.v.	Not in children
Methoxamine	5 mg i.m., i.v.	
Methyldopa	250 mg b.d. t.d.s. o. Initially 250–500 mg 6 h i.v.	10 mg/kg/day 2–4DD o. 20–40 mg/kg/day 4DD i.v.
Methylene blue	75–100 mg i.v. (1% Soln.)	
Methylphenidate	10–15 mg b.d. o. 10–20 mg s.c., i.m. i.v.	Over 6 yrs: 5–10 mg t.d.s. o Not parenteral
Methylprednisolone	Oral dose variable 16–40 mg/day, see manufacturer's literature High dose i.v.: 30 mg/kg 6 h	
Metoclopramide	5–10 mg o., i.m., i.v.	Liquid prep: 1 mg/ml Up to 1 yr: 1 mg b.d. o., i.m. 3–5 yr: 2 mg b.d. o., i.m. 6–14 yr: $2\frac{1}{2}$–5 mg t.d.s. o., i.m. *Max Dose* 0.5 mg/kg/day
Metroprolol	50 mg b.d. o. Initially 5 mg i.v. slowly. Repeat up to 15 mg	
Mexilitene	Load: 400 mg. Then 200 mg t.d.s. or q.d.s. o. 100–250 mg i.v. slowly. Infusion; 250 mg in 500 ml 0.5 mg (1 ml)/min	

Drug	Adult dose	Paediatric dose
Midazolam	0.07 mg/kg i.v., i.m.	
Minoxidil	5 mg daily o. Initially	0.2 mg/kg/day o. Max 1 mg/kg/day
Morphine	10–15 mg 4–6 h o., s.c., i.m. 5 mg i.v. Extradural and intrathecal: 2–4 mg *Preservative free* morphine *CAUTION RESPIRATORY DEPRESSION*	0.2 mg/kg i.m. 0.1 mg/kg i.v.
Nadolol	Angina: 40 mg/day o. Initially Hyperten: 80 mg/day o.	
Naloxone	0.1–0.4 mg s.c., i.m., i.v.	0.01 mg/kg i.m., i.v.
Nandrolone	25–50 mg/week i.m.	Max: 1 mg/kg/month i.m.
Nefopam	30–60 mg t.d.s. o. 20 mg 6 h i.m.	Not in children
Neostigmine	75–300 mg daily DD o. 1–2.5 mg/day DD s.c., i.m. i.v. See also anaesthetic section	Oral: Neonate 1–5 mg 4 h o. Child 15–60 mg/day DD o. Parenteral: Neonate: 50–250 μg 4 h Child: 200–500 μg/day DD
Nicotinyl alcohol	25–50 mg q.d.s. o.	Not in children
Nicoumalone	1st Day 8–12 mg o. 2nd Day 4–8 mg o. Then as per prothrombin ratio	
Nifedipine	10–20 mg t.d.s. o.	
Nikethamide	0.5–1 g i.v.	
Nitrazepam	5–10 mg nocte o.	2.5–5 mg o.
Nitroprusside	50 mg in 500 ml 5% Dextrose Infusion to control hypertension. Use drip counter and burette. *Monitor carefully.* For higher conc. see cardiac section	

10

General drugs

Drug	Adult dose	Paediatric dose
Noradrenaline	1 mg in 100 ml 5% Dextrose, rate depends on response	
Nortriptyline	10 mg q.d.s. o.	Enuresis only
Orciprenaline	1. 20 mg q.d.s. o. 2. Metered aerosol 3. 0.2 ml, 5% soln. in 2 ml by nebuliser. 4. 0.5 mg i.m.	See manufacturer's data sheet
Orphenadrine	50 mg t.d.s. o. Initially 20–40 mg i.m.	
Oubaine	0.25–0.5 mg i.v. slowly	
Oxprenolol	Angina: 40–160 mg t.d.s. o. Hyperten: 80 mg b.d. o. 2 mg i.m., i.v. slowly. Increments up to 16 mg	
Oxytocin	By infusion: 1 unit/l 1$\frac{1}{2}$-3 mUnits/min	
Papaveretum	10–20 mg 4 h i.m. 2.5 mg i.v.	0.4 mg/kg i.m.
Paracetamol	1 g q.d.s. o.	Elixir: 120 mg/5 ml 6 month–1 yr: 2.5–5 ml 1–6 yr: 5–10 ml 6–12 yr: 10–20 ml Max 4 doses in 24 h
Paraldehyde	5–10 ml i.m.	Intramuscular doses: Up to 6 months: 0.5 ml 6–12 months: 1 ml 1–2 yr: 1.5 ml 3–5 yr: 3 ml 6–12 yr: 5 ml
Penicillamine	Adult and paediatric dosage complex see manufacturers data sheet	
Pentaerythritol	30–60 mg t.d.s. o.	
Pentazocine	30–60 mg 4–6 h s.c., i.m., i.v. 50–100 mg 4 h o. 50 mg rect suppository q.d.s.	6–12 yr: 25 mg 4 h o. Max 1 mg/kg i.m. 0.5 mg/kg i.v.

Drug	Adult dose	Paediatric dose
Pentobarbitone	100–200 mg o.	
Pentolinium	Up to 10 mg i.v. in 0.5 mg increments	
Perphenazine	4 mg t.d.s. o. 5 mg 6 h i.m.	Not in children
Pethidine	50–100 mg 4 h i.m. 10–20 mg i.v. or by infusion 50–150 mg 4 h o.	1 mg/kg o. 0.5–2 mg/kg o.
Phenazocine	5 mg 4–6 h o. Max single dose 20 mg	Not in children
Phenindione	1st day: 200 mg o. 2nd day: 100 mg o. Then adjust to prothrombin ratio	
Phenobarbitone	30–60 mg t.d.s., o., i.m. 100–200 mg as hypnotic	Up to 1 year: 15–30 mg/day 1–2 years: 30–60 mg/day
Phenoperidine	1–2 mg i.v. This drug is usually administered during assisted ventilation	0.1–0.15 mg/kg i.v.
Phenoxybenzamine	10 mg b.d. o. Initially 1 mg/kg i.v. Very slowly	1–2 mg/kg/day o. 1 mg/kg i.v.
Phentolamine	Up to 10 mg i.v. in 1 mg increments Infusion: 10 mg in 100 ml, adjust rate for effect	
Phenylbutazone	200 mg t.d.s. o. Initially. Then 100 mg t.d.s. o. 250 mg nocte rect. supp.	5–10 mg/kg/day DD o.
Phenylephrine	1. Topical nasal spray 2. 100 μg i.v. 3. Infusion: 10 mg in 100 ml Adjust rate for effect	
Phenytoin	Epilepsy: 100 mg b.d.–q.d.s. o. 150–200 mg i.v. slowly or i.m. Arrhythmias: 3.5–5 mg/kg i.v.	See manufacturer's data sheet
Physostigmine	0.2–2 mg i.m., i.v.	Up to 0.03 mg/kg
Pindolol	2.5–5 mg t.d.s. o.	

10

153

General drugs

Drug	Adult dose	Paediatric dose
Piritramide	20 mg 6 h i.m.	Not in children
Piroxicam	20 mg daily o.	Not in children
Poldine	2 mg q.d.s. o.	
Practolol	5–10 mg i.v.	
Prazosin	0.5 mg b.d. or t.d.s. o. Initially	
Prednisolone	Dosage very variable see manufacturers data sheet	
Prenalterol	2.5 mg i.v. slowly. Infusion: 0.5 mg/min	
Primidone	125 mg daily o. Initially	See manufacturer's data sheet
Probenicid	250 b.d. o. Initially	Over 2 yr: 25 mg/kg 4 DD o. initially
Procainamide	250 mg 6 h o. 25 mg/min i.v. Max 1 g	
Prochlorperazine	5 mg t.d.s. o. 12.5 mg i.m.	Syrup: 5 mg in 5 ml 1–5 yr: 2.5 ml b.d. o. 6–12 yr: 5 ml b.d. or t.d.s. o.
Procyclidine	2.5 mg t.d.s. o. 5–10 mg i.v.	
Promazine	25–100 mg t.d.s. o. 50 mg 6 h i.m., i.v.	25 mg i.m. or proportional to adult dose
Promethazine	25–50 mg o., i.m.	Elixir: 5 mg in 5 ml As sedative 6 mon–1 yr: 10 mg 1–5 yr: 15–20 mg 5–10 yr: 20–25 mg i.m.: 5–10 yr 6.25–12.5 mg
Propanolol	10–40 mg t.d.s. o. 1–2 mg i.v.	0.25–1 mg/kg t.d.s. o. 0.025–0.1 mg/kg i.v.
Propantheline	15–30 mg 8 h o., i.v.	2 mg/kg/day DD max.
Protamine	1 mg neutralises 1 mg (100 units) of Heparin. Usual dose about 3 mg/kg	As adult
Protryptiline	10 mg t.d.s. o. Initially	
Pseudoephrine	60 mg t.d.s. o.	Elixir: 30 mg in 5 ml 3–12 months: 2.5 ml t.d.s. o. 1–6 yr: 5 ml t.d.s. o. 6–12 yr: 7.5 ml t.d.s. o.

Drug	Adult dose	Paediatric dose
Pyridostigmine	300 mg–1.2 g daily DD o.	Neonate: 5–10 mg 4 h o. Child: 10 mg o. initially Parenteral: Neonate 0.2–0.4 mg 4 h i.m. Child 0.25–1 mg i.m. Initially
Quinalbarbitone	50–100 mg nocte o. 200–300 mg o. for premed.	Sedation: 50–100 mg o.
Quinidine	200–400 mg b.d. o.	
Ranitidine	150 mg b.d. o. 50 mg 6–8 h i.v.	
Salbutamol	1. 4 mg q.d.s. o. 2. 0.5 mg 4 h s.c., i.m. 3. 0.25 mg i.v. slowly 4. 3–20 μg/min i.v. infusion 5. 5–10 mg of nebulised respirator soln. 6. Metered aerosol	1 Oral Syrup 2 mg in 5 ml 2–6 yr: 2.5–5 ml t.d.s. 6–12 yr: 5 ml t.d.s. 2. 2.5 mg nebulised 3. Metered aerosol 4. Not parenteral
Sotalol	80 mg b.d. o. Initially 10–20 mg i.v. slowly	
Spironolactone	100–200 mg daily o.	3 mg/kg/day DD o.
Stanozolol	5 mg daily o. 50 mg i.m. 2–3 weekly	Under 6 yr: 2.5 mg daily o. 6–10 yr: 2.5–5 mg daily o.
Streptokinase	600 000 i.u. over 30 mins i.v. 100 000 i.u. i.v. hourly for 3 days	See manufacturer's data sheet
Sulindac	200 mg b.d. o.	Not in children
Sulphasalazine	500 mg b.d.–q.d.s. o.	Reduce dose per body weight
Sulthiame	100 mg b.d. o. Initially	3–5 mg/kg/day DD o. Initially
Temazepam	10–30 mg o.	
Terbutaline	5 mg b.d. o. 0.25–0.5 mg q.d.s. s.c., i.m., i.v. slowly. Metered aerosol Ventilator nebuliser: 2–5 mg	Syrup: 0.3 mg/ml 3–7 yr: 2.5–5 ml 8 h o. 7–15 yr: 5–10 ml 8 h o. Parenteral: . 0.01 mg/kg s.c., i.m., i.v. Max. 0.3 mg
Theophylline	Several preparations with variable dosage. See manufacturer's data sheet	

10

General drugs

Drug	Adult dose	Paediatric dose
Thiethylperazine	10 mg t.d.s. o. 6.5 mg i.m. 6.5 mg rect.	Not under 15 yr
Thymoxamine	40 mg q.d.s. o. 0.1 mg/kg q.d.s. i.v.	Not in children
Thyroxine	50–100 μg daily o.	Infant: 25 μg/day then reduce Child: 2.5–5 μg/kg/day o.
Timolol	10 mg daily o.	
Tocainide	400 mg t.d.s. o. 500–750 mg i.v. slowly or infusion	
Tolbutamide	1st day – 3 g o. 2nd day – 2 g o. Maintain 1–1.5 g daily o.	Not in children
Tranexamic acid	1.5 g t.d.s. o. 500 mg–1 g i.v.	25 mg/kg/dose o. 10 mg/kg/dose i.v.
Triamcinolone	Up to 24 mg/day DD o.	
Triamterene	150–250 mg/day o.	Not in children
Triazolam	0.25 mg nocte o.	
Triclofos	1–2 g nocte o.	Up to 1 yr: 100–250 mg o. 1–5 yr: 250–500 mg o. 6–12 yr: 500 mg–1 g o.
Trifluoperazine	2–10 mg/day DD o. 1 mg i.m.	Syrup: 1 mg in 5 ml 3–5 yr: 1 mg/day DD o. 6–12 yr: 4 mg/day DD o.
Trimeprazine	10 mg t.d.s. o.	2.5–5 mg t.d.s. o. Premed: 2–4 mg/kg o.
Trimetaphan	250 mg in 500 ml 5% Dextrose infusion as required	
Trimipramine	50–75 mg nocte o.	Not in children
Triprolidine	2.5–5 mg t.d.s. o.	Elixir: 2 mg in 5 ml Up to 1 yr: 2.5 ml t.d.s. o. 1–6 yr: 5 ml t.d.s. o. 6–12 yr: 7.5 ml t.d.s. o.
Urokinase	Load: 4400 i.u./kg in 10 min Then: 4400 i.u./kg/h, infusion for 12 h	

Drug	Adult dose	Paediatric dose
Valproate sodium	600 mg/day o. Initially	Over 20 kg: 400 mg/day o. Under 20 kg: 20 mg/kg/day o.
Vasopressin	5–20 units b.d. s.c., i.m.	
Verapamil	40–120 mg t.d.s. o. 10 mg i.v. slowly and repeat 5 mg. Infusion: 5–10 mg/h. Max. 100 mg/24 h	10 mg/kg/day DD o. *Intravenous:* Infant: 0.75–2 mg 1–5 yr: 2–3 mg 6–15 yr: 2.5–5 mg
Vitamin K	10 mg i.v.	1 mg i.m., i.v.
Warfarin	10 mg, 5 mg, 5 mg, on days 1, 2 and 3. Then maintain on PTI	

10

10.4 Antibiotics

10.4.1 Introduction

This section on antibiotics is not a comprehensive guide to all
aspects of antibacterial therapy. It covers only those antibiotics
used for intensive therapy and other emergency situations in
hospital. Oral and parenteral doses are included in separate tables.
The information is basic and sufficient to initiate therapy safely. It is
not intended to replace the more detailed information available from
the manufacturer's data sheet.

Prescribing antibiotics

Antibiotics are expensive and often potentially toxic drugs, and
should only be prescribed after careful consideration. If antibiotics
are necessary, the following points should be evaluated before
giving the first dose.

Cultures of blood, sputum, urine, wound, CSF, thoracic or
abdominal drainage or other sites
Consideration of previous cultures and antibiotic sensitivity
Characteristics of the infection:
  History and possible nature
  Site
  Severity
Patient characteristics:
  Age
  Sex
  Weight
Pregnancy
Known hypersensitivity
Renal function
Hepatic function

Antibiotic Dose Tables

1. The tables
The following tables show the adult and paediatric doses of the antibiotics in common use in hospital. These doses are the normal range and unless the infection is severe the lower end of the range should be used initially. The tables are intended for reference and initiation of therapy in the absence of the manufacturer's data sheet. In severe infections much higher doses can often be used, but in these circumstances it is wise to consult a microbiologist for advice.

2. Paediatric doses
These are usually given as mg/kg/day when the total 24 h dose must be divided up as indicated. In some instances, the dose given is that actually administered at the intervals indicated.
All paediatric doses must be carefully checked before prescribing.

3. Renal Function
Most antibiotics must be given in reduced dose in the presence of any degree of renal failure, if possible, blood levels should be monitored frequently.
A detailed guide to drug therapy in renal failure can be found in the Data sheets and in the British National Formulary, pages 9–14.

4. Infusions
Detailed information about dilution and infusion of antibiotics can be found in the data sheet or in the British National Formulary.

10

5. Choice of antibiotic
Antibiotics are being developed and marketed all the time and therapeutic fashions change rapidly. It is beyond the scope of this book to recommend particular antibiotics for any but life-threatening infections when therapy cannot await results of culture and sensitivity. Under these circumstances the following combinations will cover most likely micro-organisms until cultures or microbiological advice are available.

Gentamicin, Ampicillin and Metronidazole, or
Cefotaxime and Metronidazole or, if there is a known penicillin
sensitivity:
Gentamicin and Erythromycin.
**It cannot be overemphasized that if such a policy is adopted, the
chosen drugs must be reviewed within 24 hours, when cultures, a
Gram stain, or expert advice are available.**

6. Abbreviations
Because of lack of space some abbreviations have been necessary:

mg = milligram, g = gram, kg = kilogram, 6 h = 6 hour interval
between doses, DD = Divided doses, o. = oral, i.m. =
intramuscular, i.v. = intravenous, rect. = rectal, B = Bolus
injection, usually over several minutes, I = Administration by
infusion possible or mandatory, see manufacturers literature for
details.

10.4.2 Oral Doses of antibiotics

Antibiotic	Adult oral dose	Paediatric oral dose
Amoxycillin	250–500 mg 8 h	125 mg 8 h
Amphotericin	100–200 mg 6 h (Tablets)	1 ml (100 mg) q.d.s. (Suspension)
	10 mg q.d.s. (Lozenges)	
Ampicillin	250 mg–1 g 6 h	125 mg 6 h
Cefaclor	250 mg 8 h	20 mg/kg/day DD, 8 h
Cephalexin	250–500 mg 6 h	25–50 mg/kg/day DD, 6 h
Cephradine	250–500 mg 6 h	25–50 mg/kg/day DD 6 h
Chloramphenicol	500 mg 6 h	
Cloxacillin	500 mg 6 h	1/4–1/2 Adult dose
Colistin	1.5–3 million units 8 h	Up to 15 kg:250 000–500 000 units 8 h 15–30 kg: 750 000–1 500 000 units 8 h
Co-Trimoxazole	960 mg (2 Tabs) 12 h	Paediatric Suspension: 240 mg in 5 ml 6 weeks–6 months: 2.5 ml b.d. 6 months–6 years: 5 ml b.d. 6–12 yr: 10 ml b.d.
Doxycycline	200 mg 1st day 100 mg daily	–
Erythromycin	250–500 mg 6 h	125–250 mg 6 h
Ethambutol	15 mg/kg/day	25 mg/kg/day (Reduce to 15 mg after 60 days) (see data sheet)
Flucloxacillin	250 mg 6 h	Under 2 yr: 1/4 adult dose 2–10 yr: 1/2 adult dose
Flucytosine	150–200 mg/kg/day 4DD	As adult
Isoniazid	3 mg/kg/day (max. 300 mg)	6 mg/kg/day
Kanamycin	250–500 mg 6 h	Reduce dose according to age and weight
Ketoconazole	200 mg daily	3 mg/kg/day
Metronidazole	Oral: 400 mg 8 h Rectal: 1 g 8 h	7.5 mg/kg 8 h
Miconazole	250 mg 6 h	–
Nalidixic acid	1 g 6 h	Over 3 months: 50 mg/kg/day DD
Neomycin	1 g 4 h	–

10

Antibiotics

Antibiotic	Adult oral dose	Paediatric oral dose
Nitrofurantoin	100 mg 6 h	Suspension: 25 mg/5 ml 3–30 months: 2.5 ml q.d.s. $2\frac{1}{2}$–6 yr: 5 ml q.d.s. 6–11 yr: 10 ml q.d.s. 11–14 yr: 15 ml q.d.s.
Nystatin	500 000 units 6 h (Tabs) 100 000 units 6 h (Oral susp.)	Oral susp: 100 000 units (1 ml) 6 h
Phenoxymethyl- penicillin	250–500 mg 6 h	1/4–1/2 Adult dose
Pyrazinamide	20–35 mg/kg/day 3DD	Not in children
Rifampicin	600 mg daily (10 mg/kg/day)	Up to 20 mg/kg/day (max. 600 mg/day)
Sodium fusidate	500 mg 8 h	Suspension: 175 mg/5 ml 0–1 yr: 1 ml/kg/day 3DD 1–5 yr: 5 ml t.d.s. 5–12 yr: 10 ml t.d.s.
Sulphamethizole	200 mg 5 times per day	0–5 yr: 50 mg x 5 daily 6–12 yr: 100 mg x 5 daily
Tetracycline	250–500 mg 6 h	Not in children
Tinidazole	2 g 1st day 1 g daily thereafter	Not in children under 12 yr
Trimethoprim	200 mg 12 h	2–5 months: 25 mg b.d. 6 month–5 yr: 50 mg b.d. 6–12 yr: 100 mg b.d.
Vancomycin	500 mg 6 h	44 mg/kg/day DD

10.4.3 Parenteral doses of antibiotics

Antibiotic	Adult parenteral dose	Paediatric parenteral dose
Acyclovir	5 mg/kg 8 h i.v. over 1 h	As adult
Amikacin	15 mg/kg/day 2DD i.m., i.v.,–B,I.	As adult
Amoxycillin	500 mg 8 h i.m. 1 g 6 h i.v.–B,I.	50–100 mg/kg/day DD. i.m., i.v.
Amphotericin	0.25 mg/kg/day DD i.v.-I Initially	As adult
Ampicillin	500 mg 6 h i.m., i.v.–B,I.	1/2 Adult dose
Azlocillin	Bolus i.v.: 2 g 8 h Infusion: 5 g 8 h	See manufacturer's literature
Benethamine penicillin	1 ampoule every 3 days i.m.	0–6 yr: 1/4 ampoule i.m. 7–12 yr: 1/2 ampoule i.m.
Benzylpenicillin	600 mg 6 h i.m. Up to 24 g daily by infusion - see manufacturer's literature	Neonate: 30 mg/kg/day DD, i.m. Up to 12 yr: 20 mg/kg/day DD i.m.
Carbenicillin	2 g 6 h i.m. 5 g 6 h i.v.–B,I	50–100 mg/kg/day 4DD i.m. 250–400 mg/kg/day 4DD i.v.-B,I
Cefotaxime	1 g 12 h i.m., i.v.–B,I.	100–150 mg/kg/day 4DD, i.m., i.v.
Cefoxitin	1–2 g 8 h i.m., i.v.–B,I. See manufacturer's literature	Over 3 months: 80–160 mg/kg/day 4DD i.m., i.v.
Cefsulodin	1–4 g/day 4DD i.m., i.v.-B,I	20–40 mg/kg/day DD
Ceftazidime	1–6 g/day DD i.v., i.m.	
Ceftizoxime	1–2 g 8–12 h, i.v., i.m.	Over 3 months 30–60 mg/kg/day 2–4 DD i.v., i.m.
Cefuroxime	750 mg 8 h i.m., i.v.–B.	30–100 mg/kg/day 3 DD
Cephamandole	500 mg–2 g 4–8 h i.m., i.v.–B,I.	50–100 mg/kg/day 4 DD
Cephazolin	500 mg–1 g 6–12 h i.m., i.v.–B,I.	25–50 mg/kg/day 4DD
Cephradine	500 mg–1 g 6 h i.m., i.v.–B,I.	50–100 mg/kg/day 4DD
Chloramphenicol	i.m. possible but not recommended 1 g 6–8 h i.v.–B	Infant: 25 mg/kg/day 4DD Child: 50 mg/kg/day 4DD
Cloxacillin	250 mg 6 h i.m. 500 mg 5 h i.v.–B,I.	1/4–1/2 Adult dose
Colistin	2 million units 8 h i.m., i.v.–B,I	50 000 units/kg/day 3DD

Antibiotics

Antibiotic	Adult parenteral dose	Paediatric parenteral dose
Co-Trimoxazole	960 mg (1 ampoule) 12 h i.m. 960 mg (2 ampoules) 12 h Infusion. Caution: Special preparations for i.m. and i.v. use should not be confused	See manufacturer's literature
Erythromycin	Not i.m. 600 mg 8 h i.v.–B,I	30–50 mg/kg/day 4DD i.v.-B,I.
Flucloxacillin	250 mg 6 h i.m. 250–500 mg i.v.-B,I	1/4–1/2 Adult dose
Flucytosine	150–200 mg/kg/day 4DD i.v.-I	As adult
Gentamicin	80 mg 8 h i.m., i.v.–B,I (Under 60 kg–60 mg)	Infant: 3 mg/kg 12 h i.m., i.v. Child: 2 mg/kg 8 h i.m., i.v.
Isoniazid	3 mg/kg/day i.m. (max. 300 mg) (TB meningitis: 10 mg/kg/day)	6 mg/kg/day i.m.
Kanamycin	250 mg 6 h i.m. 15–30 mg/kg/day 2 DD i.v.-I	15 mg/kg/day 2–4 DD i.m. 15–30 mg/kg/day 2–3 DD i.v.-I
Latamoxef	250 mg–3 g 12 h i.m., i.v.–B,I	Infant: 25 mg/kg 12 h Child: 50 mg/kg 12 h i.m., i.v.
Methicillin	1 g 4–6 h i.m., i.v.–B,I	Under 2 yr: 1/4 adult dose 2–10 yr: 1/2 adult dose
Metronidazole	500 mg 8 h i.v.–I Rectal: 1 g 8 h	7.5 mg/kg 8 h rect, i.v.
Mezlocillin	500 mg–2 g 6–8 h i.m. (i.v. if poss.) Bolus: 2 g 6–8 h i.v. Infusion: 5 g 6–8 h i.v.	See manufacturer's literature
Miconazole	600 mg 8 h i.v.–I	40 mg/kg/day DD
Netilmicin	4–6 mg/kg/day DD 12 h i.m., i.v.–B,I	Neonate: 6 mg/kg/day DD 12 h Infant: 7.5–9 mg/kg/day DD 12 h Child: 6–7.5 mg/kg/day DD 12 h
Piperacillin	100–150 mg/kg/day 4DD i.m., i.v.-B,I	Infant: 100–300 mg/kg/day 2DD Child: 100–300 mg/kg/day 3DD

Antibiotic	Adult parenteral dose	Paediatric parenteral dose
Procaine penicillin	300 mg 12 h i.m.	Reduce dose proportionally under 25 kg
Rifampicin	In severe infections an intravenous preparation is available at special request	
Sodium fusidate	500 mg infusion over 6 h at 8–hourly intervals	Under 50 kg: 6–7 mg/kg 8 h by infusion i.v. over 6 h
Streptomycin	1 g daily i.m. (750 mg over 40 yr)	30 mg/kg daily i.m. (max. 1 g)
Tetracycline	100 mg 8 h i.m. 500 mg 12 h i.v.–I	Not in children
Ticarcillin	15–20 g/day 4DD i.m., i.v.–B,I	200–300 mg/kg/day 4DD
Tinidazole	800 mg daily i.v. –I	Not in children
Tobramycin	3–5 mg/kg/day DD 8 h i.m., i.v.–B,I	Infant: 4 mg/kg/day DD 12 h Child: 6 mg/kg/day DD 6 h
Trimethoprim	150–250 mg 12 h i.v.–B,I	Under 12 yr: 8 mg/kg/day 3DD i.v.
Vancomycin	500 mg 6 h i.v.–I	44 mg/kg/day 4 DD i.v.-I

10

10.5 Brand names to pharmacopoeal names conversion

Brand Name	Pharmacopoeal name	Brand name	Pharmacopoeal name
Achromycin	—tetracycline	Arvin	—ancrod
Acthar	—ACTH	Asendin	—amoxapine
Actifed	—trypolikine	Atarax	—hydroxyzine
Adalat	—nifedipine	Ativan	—lorazepam
Adapin	—doxepin	Atromid–S	—clofibrate
Adriamycin	—doxorubicin	Atrovent	—ipratropium
Aerolate	—theophylline	Aventyl	—nortryptyline
Afrinol	—pseudoephedrine	Avomine	—promethazine
Alcobon	—flucytosine	Azapen	—methicillin
Aldactone	—spironolactone	Azolid	—phenylbutazone
Aldomet	—methyl dopa		
Algodex	—propoxyphene	Bactopen	—cloxacillin
Allegron	—nortryptiline	Bactrim	—trimethaprim +
Alloferin	—alcuronium		sulphamexazole
Alpen–N	—ampicillin	Banlin	—propantheline
Alupent	—metaproterenol	Baratol	—indoramin
Alupent	—orciprenaline	Brypen	—mezlocillin
Amicar	—aminocaproic acid	Benadryl	—diphenhydramine
Amikin	—amikacin	Bendylate	—diphenhydramine
Amiline	—amitryptiline	Benemid	—probenecid
Amisec	—aminophylline	Bentyl	—dicyclomine
Amitid	—amitriptyline	Berkdopa	—levodopa
Amoxil	—amoxicillin	Berkfurin	—nitrofurantoin
Amphicol	—chloramphenicol	Berkozide	—bendrofluazide
Ampifen	—ampicillin	Beta-Cardone	—sotalol
Ampilean	—ampicillin	Betaloc	—metoprolol
Amytal	—amylobarbitone	Betim	—timolol
Anafranil	—clomipramine	Betnesol	—betamethasone
Anectine	—suxamethonium	Bicillin	—procaine penicillin
Ansolysen	—pentolinium	Bio-Tetra	—tetracycline
Anthisan	—mepyramine	Biogastrone	—carbenoxalone
Antilirium	—physostigmine	Bisolvon	—bromhexine
Antipress	—imipramine	Blocadren	—timolol
Apogen	—gentamicin	Bretylate	—bretylium tosilate
Apresoline	—hydralazine	Brevidil-M	—suxamethonium
Aprinox	—bendrofluazide	Bricanyl	—terbutaline
Apsin	—phenoxymethylpenicillin	Brietal	—methohexitone
Apsolox	—oxprenolol	Brocadopa	—levodopa
Aquastat	—benzthiazide	Burinex	—bumetanide
Aralen	—chloroquine	Buscopan	—hyoscine
Aramine	—metaraminol	Butacote	—phenylbutazone
Arfonad	—trimetaphan	Butazolidine	—phenylbutazone
Aristogel	—triamcinolone		

Brand names to pharmacopoeal names conversion

Brand name	Pharmacopoeal name	Brand name	Pharmacopoeal name
Cafergot	—ergotamine + caffeine	Cordarone	—amiodarone
Calan	—verapamil	Cordilox	—verapamil
Calpol	—paracetamol	Corgard	—nadolol
Campain	—acetaminophen	Coronex	—isosorbide dinitrate
Caplenal	—allopurinol	Corophyllin	—aminophylline
Capoten	—captopril	Cortelan	—cortisone
Carbacel	—carbachol	Cortisporin	—neomycin
Cardiacap	—pentaerythritol	Cortistab	—cortisone
Cardilate	—erythrityl tetranitrate	Cortisyl	—cortisone
Cardioquin	—quinidine	Cortogen	—cortisone
Catapres	—clonidine	Crystapen V	—phenoxymethylpenicillin
Ceclor	—cefaclor	Crystapen	—benzylpenicillin
Cedinalid	—lanatoside-C	Crystodigin	—digitoxin
Cedocard	—isosorbide	Cuprimine	—penicillamine
Cefizox	—ceftizoxime	Cyantin	—nitrofurantoin
Celbenin	—methicillin	Cyclimorph	—morphine + cyclizine
Celestone	—betamethasone	Cyclobral	—cyclandelate
Centyl	—bendrofluazide	Cyclokapron	—tranexamic acid
Ceporex	—cephalexin	Cyclospasmol	—cyclandelate
Cerebid	—papaverine	Cytacon	—cyanocobalamin
Chloralex	—chloral hydrate	Cytamen	—cyanocobalamin
Chloramate	—chlorpheniramine	Cytoxan	—cyclophosphamide
Chloramead	—chlorpromazine		
Chlorocain	—mepivicaine	Daktarin	—miconazole
Chloromide	—chlorpropamide	Dalmane	—flurazepam
Chloromycetin	—chloramphenicol	Dantoin	—phenytoin
Choledyl	—choline theophyllinate	Dantrium	—dantrolene
Chymar	—chymotrypsin	Daonil	—glibenclamide
Chymoral	—chymotrypsin	Darvon	—propoxyphene
Cidomycin	—gentamicin	Debendox	—dicyclomine
Citanest	—prilocaine	Decadron	—dexamethasone
Claforan	—cefotaxime	Declinax	—debrisoquine
Clairvan	—ethamivan	Deltasone	—prednisolone
Claripex	—clofibrate	Demerol	—pethidine
Cleocin	—clindamycin	Dendrid	—idoxuridine
Clinazine	—trifluoperazine	Depen	—penicillamine
Clinoral	—sulindac	Depo-Medrone	—methylprednisolone
Clonoral	—sulindac	Depocillin	—procaine penicillin
Co-Betaloc	—metoprolol	Desferal	—desferrioxamine
Cogentin	—benziropine	Desoxyn	—methamphetamine
Colomycin	—colistin	Dexedrine	—dexamphetamine
Compazine	—prochlorperazine	DF118	—dihydrocodeine
Concordin	—protryptiline	Diabenese	—chlorpropamide
Contac	—phenylephrine		

10

Brand names to pharmacopoeal names conversion

Brand name	Pharmacopoeal name	Brand name	Pharmacopoeal name
Diamox	—acetazolamide	Elavil	—amitriptyline
Diatensec	—spirolonactone	Emeside	—ethsuximide
Diazemuls	—valium	Epanutin	—phenytoin
Diazide	—triamterine	Epilim	—sodium valproate
Dibenyline	—phenoxybenzamine	Epinephrine	—adrenaline
Dibucaine	—nupercaine	Epontol	—propanidid
Diconal	—dipipanone	Epsicapron	—aminocaproic acid
Dicynene	—ethamsylate	Equanil	—meprobamate
Dilantin	—phenytoin	Eraldin	—practolol
Dimelor	—acetohexamide	Ergotrate	—ergometrine
Dindevan	—phenindione	Erycen	—erythromycin
Dipidolor	—piritramide	Erythrocin	—erythromycin
Disipal	—orphenadrine	Erythromid	—erythromycin
Distaclor	—cefaclor	Erythroped	—erythromycin
Distalgaesic	—dextropropoxephene	Esbatal	—bethanidine
Distamine	—penicillamine	Esidrex	—hydrochlorthiazide
Distaquaine	—phenoxymethylpenicillin	Eskabarb	—phenobarbitone
Diumide	—frusemide	Ethrane	—enflurane
Diuril	—chlorthiazide	Etophylate	—acepifylline
Dixarit	—clonidine	Eudemine	—diazoxide
Dobutrex	—dobutamine	Euglucon	—clibenclamide
Dolobid	—diflunisal	Euhypnos	—temazepam
Doloxene	—dextropropoxyphene	Eulissin	—decamethonium
Dopamet	—methyl dopa	Eumydrin	—atropine methonitrate
Dopram	—doxapram	Eutonyl	—pargyline
Doriden	—glutethamide		
Doryl	—carbachol	F-Cortef	—fludrocortisone
Dramamine	—dimenhydrinate	Fasigyn	—tinidazole
Droleptan	—droperidol	Fazadon	—fazadinium
Dromoran	—levorphanol	Feldene	—piroxicam
Dryptal	—frusemide	Femergin	—ergotamine tartrate
Duogastrone	—carbenoxalone	Fenopron	—fenoprofen
Duphalac	—lactulose	Fentazin	—perphenazine
Durabolin	—nandrolone	Flagyl	—metronidazole
Duranest	—etidocaine	Flaxedil	—gallamine
Duvalidan	—isoxsuprine	Flexon	—orphenadrine
Dyrenium	—triamterine	Florinef	—fludrocortisone
Dytac	—triamterine	Floxapen	—flucloxacillin
		Fluothane	—halothane
EACA	—aminocaproic acid	Folvite	—folic acid
Edecrin	—ethacrynic acid	Fomac	—salicylic acid
Efcortelan	—hydrocortisone	Fortagaesic	—pentazocine +
Effergot	—ergotamine		paracetamol

Brand names to pharmacopoeal names conversion

Brand name	Pharmacopoeal name	Brand name	Pharmacopoeal name
Fortral	—pentazocine	Ilosin	—erythromycin
Fortum	—ceftazidime	Imferon	—iron dextran
Franol	—ephedrine	Imodium	—loperamide
Frisium	—clobazam	Imuran	—azothioprine
Froben	—fluriprofen	Inapsine	—droperidol
Fucidin	—fusidic acid	Inderal	—propanolol
Fungilin	—amphotericin	Indocid	—indomethacin
Furadantin	—nitrofurantoin	Indon	—phenindione
Furosemide	—frusemide	Innovar	—droperidol/fentanyl
		Intal	—sodium chromo-
Garamycin	—gentamicin		glycate
Gardenal	—phenobarbitone	Intraval	—thiopentone
Genticin	—gentamicin	Intropin	—dopamine
Gentisone	—gentamicin	Inversine	—mecamylamine
Geocillin	—carbenicillin	Ipral	—trimethoprim
Glucophage	—metformin	Ismelin	—guanethidine
Gynergan	—ergotamine tartrate	Isobarb	—pentobarbitone
		Isobec	—amylobarbitone
Halcion	—triazolam	Isofedrol	—ephedrine
Haldol	—haloperidol	Isoproterenol	—isoprenaline
Hedulin	—phenindione	Isoptin	—verapamil
Heminevrin	—chlormethiazole	Isordil	—isosorbide
Hepacon	—cyanocobalamin		
Heroin	—diamorphine	Kabikinase	—streptokinase
Herpid	—idoxuridine	Kannasyn	—kanamycin
Hexopal	—inositol	Kanterx	—kanamycin
Histalon	—chlorpheniramine	Kaomycin	—neomycin
Hyalase	—hyaluronidase	Kefadol	—cephamandole
Hydergine	—co-dergocrine	Keflex	—cephalexin
Hydrocortone	—hydrocortisone	Kefzol	—cephazolin
Hydromet	—methyl dopa	Kemadrin	—procyclidine
Hydrosaluric	—hydrochlorthiazide	Kemicetine	—chloramphenicol
Hygroton	—chlorthalidone	Kenolog	—triamcinolone
Hyperstat	—diazoxide	Ketelar	—ketamine
Hypnomidate	—etomidate	Kinidin	—quinidine
Hypnovel	—midazolam	Konakion	—vitamin K
Hypon	—aspirin/caffeine/	Korostatin	—nystatin
	codeine		
Hypovase	—prazosin	Labophylline	—theophylline
Hyprenan	—prenalterol	Lanitop	—medigoxin
Hypurin	—insulin	Lanvis	—thioguanine
Hyzazyme	—hyaluronidase	Largactil	—chlorpromazine
		Larodopa	—levodopa
Iletin	—insulin		

10

Brand name	Pharmacopoeal name	Brand name	Pharmacopoeal name
Larotid	—amoxicillin	Metaproteren	—orciprenaline
Lasix	—frusemide	Methadrine	—methyl-amphetamine
Ledercort	—triamcinolone	Mexitil	—mexilitine
Lederfen	—fenbufen	Mictral	—nalidixic acid
Ledermycin	—demeclocycline	Midamor	—amiloride
Lentizol	—amitryptiline	Migril	—ergotamine tartrate
Lethidrone	—nalorphine	Miltown	—meprobamate
Leucovorin	—calcium folinate	Miochol	—acetylcholine
Leukeran	—chlorambucil	Mistostat	—carbachol
Levarterenol	—noradrenaline	Mobenol	—tolbutamide
Levophed	—noradrenaline	Moctamid	—lormetazepam
Libraxin	—chlordiazepoxide	Modecate	—fluphenazine
Lidocaine	—lignocaine	Moditen	—fluphenazine
Limbritol	—amitryptiline	Moducren	—amiloride
Lingraine	—ergotamine	Moduretic	—amiloride
Liskonum	—lithium	Mogadon	—nitrazepam
Litarex	—lithium	Monaspor	—cefsulodin
Lomotil	—diphenoxylate + atropine	Monistat	—miconazole
Lopressor	—metoprolol	Monotrim	—trimethoprim
Lopurin	—allopurinol	Motipress	—fluphenazine
Lorfan	—levallorphan	Moxalactam	—latamoxef
Luminal	—phenobarbitone	Murcil	—chlordiazepoxide
		Myambutol	—ethambutol
Macrodantin	—nitrofurantoin	Myanesin	—mephenesin
Madopar	—levodopa/benserazide	Mycardol	—pentaerythritol
Magnapen	—ampicillin/flucloxacillin	Myleran	—bulsulphan
Maladrin	—ephedrine	Mynah	—ethambutol/isoniazid
Marcain	—bupivicaine	Mysoline	—primidone
Marevan	—warfarin	Mystereclin	—tetracycline
Marezine	—cyclizine		
Marplan	—isocarboxazid		
Marsilid	—iproniazid	Nacton	—poldine
Maxalon	—metoclopramide	Nandrolone	—durabolin
Medrone	—methylprednisolone	Naprosyn	—naproxen
Mefoxin	—cefoxitin	Napsalgaesic	—dextropropoxyphene
Melitase	—chlorpropamide	Narcan	—phenazocine
Melleril	—thioridazine	Narphan	—phenazocine
Menandione	—vitamin K	Naturetin	—bendrofluazide
Meperidine	—pethidine	Navidrex	—cyclopenthiazide
Mephine	—mephentermine	Nebcin	—tobramycin
Meptid	—meptazinol	Negram	—naledixic acid
Meravil	—amitriptyline	Nemasol	—aminosalicylate
Mestinon	—pyridostigmine	Nembutal	—pentobarbitone
Mesylate	—phentolamine	Neomercazole	—carbimazole

Brand names to pharmacopoeal names conversion

Brand name	Pharmacopoeal name	Brand name	Pharmacopoeal name
Neonaclex	— bendrofluazide	Parest	— methaqualone
Neosporin	— polymyxin	Pavulon	— pancuronium
Neosynephrine	— phenylephrine	Penamox	— amoxicillin
Neticillin	— netilmicin	Penbritin	— ampicillin
Neuphane	— isophane insulin	Pendramine	— penicillamine
Nipride	— nitroprusside	Penthrane	— methoxyflurane
Nitrados	— nitrazepam	Pentothal	— thiopentone
Nitrocontin	— glyceryl trinitrate	Percutol	— glyceryl trinitrate
Nitrolingual	— glyceryl trinitrate	Pethilorphan	— pethidine/levallorphan
Nivemycin	— neomycin	Phenergan	— promethazine
Nizoral	— ketoconazole	Physeptone	— methadone
Nobrium	— medazepam	Pipril	— piperacillin
Noctamid	— lormetazepam	Piriton	— chlorpheniramine
Noctec	— chloral hydrate	Pitocin	— oxytocin
Nodilon	— co-trimoxazole	Pitressin	— vasopressin
Norcuron	— vecuronium	Polycillin	— ampicillin
Norflex	— orphenadrine	Ponstan	— mefenamic acid
Normison	— temazepam	Ponstel	— mefenamic acid
Norpace	— disopyramide	Pontocaine	— amethocaine
Norpramin	— desipramine	Pramidex	— tolbutamide
Novocaine	— procaine	Primperan	— metoclopramide
Novopen	— penicillin	Prindalol	— phenazocine
Novosemide	— frusemide	Priscol	— tolazoline
Nu-Seals	— aspirin	Probanthine	— propantheline
Nupercaine	— cinchocaine	Probesic	— fenoprofen
Nydrazix	— isoniazid	Proglycem	— diazoxide
Nystan	— nystatin	Pronestyl	— procainamide
		Propitocaine	— prilocaine
Oblivon	— methylpentinol	Prostigmine	— neostigmine
Obracin	— tobramycin	Proternol	— isoprenaline
Omnipen	— ampicillin	Proventil	— albuterol
Omnopon	— papaveretum	Pularin	— heparin
Operidine	— phenoperidine	Pyopen	— carbenicillin
Opilon	— thymoxamine		
Orbenin	— cloxacillin	Rastinon	— tolbutamide
Ospolot	— sulthiame	Regitine	— phentolamine
		Reglan	— metoclopramide
Palaprin	— aloxiprin (aspirin)	Reposans	— chlordiazepoxide
Palfium	— dextromoramide	Restoril	— temazepam
Panadol	— paracetamol	Rhythmodan	— disopyramide
Panheprin	— heparin	Rifaden	— rifampicin
Paracodin	— dihydrocodin	Rifapen	— alfentanil
Parasal	— aminosalicylic acid	Rimafon	— isoniazid

10

171

Brand names to pharmacopoeal names conversion

Brand name	Pharmacopoeal name	Brand name	Pharmacopoeal name
Ritalin	—methylphenidate	Stelazine	—trifluperazine
Rivotril	—clonazepam	Stemetil	—prochlorperazine
Robamox	—amoxicillin	Stromba	—stanozolol
Robinul	—glycopyrronium	Strophanthin G	—ouabaine
Rogitine	—phentolamine	Strycin	—streptomycin
Rohypnol	—flunitrazepam	Stugeron	—cinnarizine
Rolazine	—hydralazine	Sublimase	—pseudoephedrine
Ronicol	—nicotinyl alcohol	Sulphasalazine	—salazopyrin
Rougoxin	—digoxin	Surem	—nitrazepam
		Surmontil	—trimipramine
Salazopyrin	—sulphasalazine	Sustac	—glyceryl trinitrate
Saluric	—chlorthiazide	Symcurin	—decamethonium
Saventrine	—isoprenaline	Symmetril	—amantadine
Scoline	—suxamethonium	Syndol	—paracetamol/codeine/
Scopolamine	—hyoscine		doxylamine
Seconal	—quinalbarbitone	Synkavit	—menadiol
Sectral	—acebutolol	Syntocinon	—oxytocin
Securopen	—azlocillin	Syraprim	—trimethoprim
Seominal	—phenobarbitone/theo-		
	bromine	Tacrine	—tetrahydroaminoacridine
Septrin	—trimethoprim + sulpha-	Tagamet	—cimetidine
	methoxazole	Talwin	—pentazocine
Serax	—oxazepam	Tedral	—theophylline/ephedrine
Serenace	—haloperidol	Tegretol	—carbamazepine
Serenid	—oxazepam	Teldrin	—chlorpheniramine
Serpasil	—reserpine	Temaril	—trimeprazine
Silbephylline	—diprophylline	Temgesic	—buprenorphine
Sinemet	—laevodopa	Tenormin	—atenolol
Sinequan	—doxepin	Tensilon	—edrephonium
Sinthrome	—nicoumalone	Tenuate Dospan	—diethylpropion
Sodium amytal	—sodium amylobarbitone	Tetracaine	—amethocaine
Solumedrone	—methylprednisolone	Tetracyn	—tetracycline
Somnite	—nitrazepam	Thalamonal	—droperidol/fentanyl
Somnos	—chloral hydrate	Thalazole	—phthalylsulphathiazole
Soneryl	—butobarbitone	Theograd	—theophylline
Sonislo	—isosorbide	Thorazine	—chlorpromazine
Sorbid	—isosorbide	Ticar	—ticarcillin
Sorbitrate	—isosorbide	Timoptol	—timolol
Sotacor	—sotalol	Tofranil	—imipramine
Sparine	—promazine	Tolserol	—mephenesin
Spiroctan	—spironolactone	Tonocard	—tocainide
Stabinol	—chlorpropamide	Torecan	—thiethylperazine

Brand names to pharmacopoeal names conversion

Brand name	Pharmacopoeal name	Brand name	Pharmacopoeal name
Tracrium	—atracurium	Varidase	—streptokinase
Trancopal	—chlormezanone	Vascardin	—isosorbide
Trandate	—labetolol	Vasculite	—bamethan
Tranmep	—meprobamate	Vasoxine	—methoxamine
Tranxene	—chlorazepate	Vasoxyl	—methoxamine
Trasicor	—oxprenolol	Vatensol	—guanoclor
Trental	—oxpentifylline	Veganin	—aspirin/paracetamol/
Trichloryl	—triclofos		codeine
Tridil	—glyceryl trinitrate	Velbe	—vinblastin
Tridione	—troxidone	Velosef	—cephradine
Triflurin	—trifluoperazine	Ventolin	—salbutamol
Trilafon	—perfenazine	Veriloid	—veratrum
Trilene	—trichlorethylene	Vertigon	—prochlorperazine
Trimopan	—trimethoprim	Vibramycin	—doxycycline
Triptafen	—amitryptiline	Vidopen	—ampicillin
Tubarine	—tubocurarine	Visken	—pindolol
Tuinal	—quinal+amylobarbitone	Vistaril	—hydroxyzine
		Vivol	—diazepam
Ubretid	—distigmine	Voltarol	—diclofenac
Ukidan	—urokinase		
Unigesid	—paracetamol	Warnerin	—warfarin
Uridon	—chlorthalidone	Welldorm	—dichlorphenazone
Urispas	—flavoxate	Wyamine	—mephentermine
Uritol	—frusemide		
Urizide	—bendrofluazide	Xseb	—salicylic acid
Urolucosil	—sulphamethazole	Xylocaine	—lignocaine
Uromide	—sulphacarbamide		
Urozide	—hydrochlorthiazide	Zantac	—ranitidine
Uticillin	—carfecillin	Zarontin	—ethosuxamide
		Zetran	—chlordiazepoxide
Valium	—diazepam	Zinacef	—cefuroxime
Vallergan	—trimeprazine	Zinamide	—pyrazinamide
Valoid	—cyclizine	Zovirax	—acyclovir
Vancocin	—vancomycin	Zyloric	—allopurinol

10

10.6 Drug interactions

'Drug 1' and 'Drug 2' are the columns containing the two drugs to be mixed. Column 3 shows the effect of mixing these drugs.

Drug 1	Drug 2	Effect
Acetohexamide	Phenylbutazone	Hypoglycaemia
Alcohol	Barbiturates	Potentiation of barbiturates
	General anaesthetics	Potentiation of GA's
	Phenothiazines	Potentiation of phenothiazines
Allopurinol	6-Mercaptopurine	Increased cytotoxic effects
	Azathioprine	Increased cytotoxic effects
Amphetamines	Antihypertensives	Reversal of antihypertensive effect
	Barbiturates	Altered CNS effects
	Ganglion blockers	Reversal of hypotension
	MAOI's	Hypertensive crises
Anabolic steriods	Anticoagulants	Increased anticoagulant effect
Anaesthetics	Guanethidine	Hypotension
	Methyl dopa	Hypotension
	Reserpine	Hypotension
Analeptics	MAOI's	CNS stimulation
Anticholinesterases	Curareform relaxants	Reversal of relaxants
Anticoagulant	Barbiturates	Potentiation of barbiturates
	'Mycin' antibiotics	Potentiation of anticoagulants
	Anabolic steriods	Increased anticoagulant effect
	Barbiturates	Reduced anticoagulant effect
	Chloral Hydrate	Increased anticoagulant effect
	Clofibrate	Increased anticoagulant effect
	Salicylates	Increased anticoagulant effect
	Tolbutamide	Hypoglycaemia
	Vitamin K	Reduced anticoagulant effect
Antihypertensives	Amphetamines	Reversal of antihypertensive effect
	Ganglion blockers	Increased hypotension
Antiparkinsonism drugs	MAOI's	CNS stimulation
Antithyroid drugs	Benzodiazepines	Increased antithyroid effect
Azathioprine	Allopurinol	Increased cytotoxic effects
Barbiturates	Alcohol	Potentiation of barbiturates
	Amphetamines	Altered CNS effect
	Anticoagulants	Reduced anticoagulant effect
	Contraceptives	Reduced contraceptive reliability
	Griseofulvin	Reduced antibiotic effect
	Ketamine	Chemically incompatible
	Quinidine	Quinidine action reduced
	Steroids	Hyposteroid crisis in dependant patients
	Suxamethonium	Reduced effect of suxamethonium
Benzodiazepines	Antithyroid drugs	Increased antithyroid effect

Drug 1	Drug 2	Effect
Beta blockers	Cyclopropane	Potentiation of cyclopropane
	Ketamine	Potentiation of ketamine
Bilirubin	Pyrazolones	Raised bilirubin
	Salicylates	Raised bilirubin
	Sulphonamides	Raised bilirubin
Caffeine	Hypnotics	Hypnosis antagonized
Calcium	Digoxin	Enhances dysrhythmias
Catecholamines	Tricyclic antidepressants	Hypertension
	Halothane	Dysrhythmias
Cephalosporins	Probenecid	Raised levels of cephalosporins
Chloral hydrate	Anticoagulants	Increased anticoagulant effect
Chloramphenicol	Phenytoin	Increased phenytoin levels
Clofibrate	Anticoagulants	Increased anticoagulant effect
CNS depressants	CNS depressants	Enhanced depression, drowsiness
Contraceptives	Barbiturates	Reduced contraceptive reliability
	Phenytoin	Reduced contraceptive reliability
Corticosteroids	Phenytoin	Corticosteroid effect reduced
Curareform relaxants	Anticholinesterases	Reversal of relaxants
	Halothane	Increased hypotension
	Mycin antibiotics	Potentiation of relaxants
	Thiazides	Prolonged relaxation
Cyclopropane	Beta blockers	Potentiation of cyclopropane
Cytotoxics	Suxamethonium	Prolonged apnoea
Digoxin	Calcium	Enhances dysrhythmias
	Diuretics	Potentiation of digoxin
	Propantheline	Reduced absorption due to low gut motility
	Reserpines	Bradycardia
	Suxamethonium	Enhanced digoxin toxicity
Disulphiram	Phenytoin	Increased phenytoin levels
	Warfarin	Increased warfarin levels
Diuretics	Digoxin	Potentiation of digoxin
	Ganglion blockers	Potentiation of ganglion blockers
	Guanethidine	Hypotension
	MAOI's	Increased hypertension
	Methyl dopa	Hypotension
	Reserpine	Hypotension
	Suxamethonium	Increase in potassium
Dyflos	Suxamethonium	Potention of relaxants
Ecothiopate	Suxamethonium	Enhanced neuromuscular blockade
Ganglion blockers	Amphetamines	Reversal of hypotension
	Antihypertensives	Increased hypotension
	Diuretics	Potentiation of ganglion blockers
	MAOI's	Hypotension

10

Drug interactions

Drug 1	Drug 2	Effect
Ganglion blockers	Phenothiazines	Increased effect of ganglion blockers
	Tricyclic antidepres-sants	Reversal of hypotension
General anaesthetics	Alcohol	Potentiation of GA's
Glutethamide	Steroids	Hyposteroid crisis in dependant patients
Griseofulvin	Barbiturates	Reduced antibiotic effect
Guanethidine	Anaesthetics	Hypotension
	Diuretics	Hypotension
	Sympathomimetics	Hypertension
	Tricyclic antidepres-sants	Reduced hypotensive effect
Halothane	Catecholamines	Dysrhythmias
	Curareform relaxants	Increased hypotension
	Levodopa	Hypertension vasoconstriction
Heparin	Penicillin	Chemically incompatible
	Protamine	Antagonistic
	Steroids	Chemically incompatible
Hypnotics	Caffeine	Hypnosis antagonized
Indomethacin	Probenecid	Raised levels of indomethacin
Insulin	Propanolol	Hypoglycaemia
	Salicylates	Hypoglycaemia
Iron	Tetracyclines	Reduced absorption of antibiotics
Ketamine	Barbiturates	Chemically incompatible
	Beta blockers	Potentiation of ketamine
Levodopa	Halothane	Hypertension
MAOI's	Amphetamines	Hypertensive crises
	Analeptics	CNS stimulation
	Antiparkinsonism drugs	CNS stimulation
	Diuretics	Increased hypertension
	Ganglion blockers	Hypotension
	Opiates	Potentiation of opiates
	Phenylephrine	Potentiation of phenylephrine
	Sulphonyl ureas	Hypoglycaemia
	Tricyclic antidepres-sants	Potentiation of antidepressant effect
Methotrexate	Salicylates	Increased cytotoxic effects
Methyl dopa	Anaesthetics	Hypotension
	Diuretics	Hypotension
	Sympathomimetics	Reduced hypotensive effect
	Tricyclic antidepres-sants	Reduced hypotensive effect

Drug 1	Drug 2	Effect
Mycin antibiotics	Anticoagulants	Potentiation of anticoagulants
	Curareform relaxants	Potentiation of relaxants
	Muscle relaxants	Potentiation of relaxation
Nalidixic acid	Probenecid	Raised levels of nalidixic acid
Naloxone	Opiate	Reversal of opiate effect
Nephrotoxic drugs	Nephrotoxic drugs	Enhancement of effect
Opiates	MAOI's	Potentiation of opiates
	Naloxone	Reversal of opiate effect
	Pentazocine	Reduced opiate effect
PABA local anaesthetics	Sulphonamides	Reduced antimicrobial effects
Penicillin	Heparin	Chemically incompatible
	Probenecid	Raised levels of penicillins
Pentazocine	Opiates	Reduced opiate effect
Phenothiazines	Alcohol	Potentiation of phenothiazines
	Ganglion blockers	Increased effect of ganglion blockers
	Steroids	Hyposteroid crisis in dependant patients
Phenylbutazone	Acetohexamide	Hypoglycaemia
Phenylephrine	MAOI's	Potentiation of phenylephrine
Phenytoin	Chloramphenicol	Increased phenytoin levels
	Contraceptives	Reduced contraceptive reliability
	Corticosteroids	Corticosteroid effect reduced
	Disulphiram	Increased phenytoin levels
	Pyrazolones	Potentiation of phenytoin
	Steroids	Hyposteroid crisis in dependant patients
	Sulphonamides	Potentiation of phenytoin
Physostigmine	Suxamethonium	Potentiation of relaxant
Probenecid	Cephalosporins	Raised levels of cephalosporins
	Indomethacin	Raised levels of indomethacin
	Nalidixic Acid	Raised levels of nalidixic acid
	Penicillins	Raised levels of penicillins
	Salicylates	Antagonism of uricosuric effect
Procaine	Suxamethonium	Prolonged relaxation
Propanidid	Suxamethonium	Prolonged apnoea
Propanolol	Insulin	Hypoglycaemia
	Sulphonyl ureas	Hypoglycaemia
Propantheline	Digoxin	Reduced absorption due to low gut motility
Protamine	Heparin	Antagonistic
Pyrazolones	Bilirubin	Raised bilirubin
	Phenytoin	Potentiation of phenytoin
	Sulphonyl ureas	Hypoglycaemia
Pyridostigmine	Suxamethonium	Potentiation of relaxant

10

177

Drug interactions

Drug 1	Drug 2	Effect
Quinidine	Barbiturate	Quinidine action reduced
Reserpine	Anaesthetics	Hypotension
	Diuretics	Hypotension
	Sympathomimetics	Hypertension
	Tricyclic antidepres-sants	Reduced hypotensive effect
	Digoxin	Bradycardia
Salicylates	Anticoagulants	Increased anticoagulant effect
	Bilirubin	Raised bilirubin
	Insulin	Hypoglycaemia
	Methotrexate	Increased cytotoxic effects
	Probenecid	Antagonism of uricosuric effect
	Sulphonamides	Increased antibiotic effect
	Sulphonyl ureas	Hypoglycaemia
Six mercaptopurine	Allopurinol	Increased cytotoxic effects
Steroids	Barbiturates	Hyposteroid crisis in dependant patients
	Glutethamide	Hyposteroid crisis in dependant patients
	Heparin	Chemically incompatible
	Phenothiazines	Hyposteroid crisis in dependant patients
	Phenytoin	Hyposteroid crisis in dependant patients
	Thiazides	Hyperglycaemia
	Tricyclic antidepres-sants	Chemically incompatible
Sulphafurazole	Thiopentone	Increased effect of thiopentone
Sulphonamides	Bilirubin	Raised bilirubin
	PABA Local Anaes-thetics	Reduced antimicrobial effects
	Phenytoin	Potentiation of phenytoin
	Salicylates	Increased antibiotic effect
	Sulphonyl ureas	Hypoglycaemia
Sulphonyl Ureas	MAOI's	Hypoglycaemia
	Propanolol	Hypoglycaemia
	Pyrazolones	Hypoglycaemia
	Salicylates	Hypoglycaemia
	Sulphonamides	Hypoglycaemia
Suxamethonium	Barbiturates	Reduced effect of suxamethonium
	Cytotoxics	Prolonged apnoea
	Digoxin	Enhanced digoxin toxicity
	Diuretics	Increase in potassium
	Dyflos	Potentiation of relaxants
	Ecothiopate	Enhanced neuromuscular blockade
	Physostigmine	Potentiation of relaxant
	Procaine	Prolonged relaxation
	Propanidid	Prolonged apnoea
	Pyridostigmine	Potentiation of relaxant

Drug 1	Drug 2	Effect
Suxamethonium	Trifluperazine	Reduced effect of suxamethonium
Sympathomimetics	Guanethidine	Hypertension
	Methyl dopa	Reduced hypotensive effect
	Reserpine	Hypertension
Tetracyclines	Iron	Reduced absorption of antibiotics
Thiazides	Curareform relaxants	Prolonged relaxation
	Steroids	Hyperglycaemia
Thiopentone	Sulphafurazole	Increased effect of thiopentone
Tolbutamide	Anticoagulants	Hypoglycaemia
Tricyclic antidepressants	Catecholamines	Hypertension
	Ganglion blockers	Reversal of hypotension
	Guanethidine	Reduced hypotensive effects
	MAOI's	Potentiation of antidepressant effect
	Methyl dopa	Reduced hypotensive effect
	Reserpine	Reduced hypotensive effect
	Steroids	Chemically incompatible
Trifluperazine	Suxamethonium	Reduced effect of suxamethonium
Vitamin K	Anticoagulants	Decreased anticoagulant effect
Warfarin	Disulphiram	Increased warfarin levels

10

SECTION 11
RENAL FAILURE

11

11.1 Renal failure diagnosis

Urine	Renal	Prerenal	Normal
Osmolality	285–295	<400	400–1400
Response to Lasix 500 mg	Poor	Fair	Very good
Blood/urine urea ratio	<5:1	<10:1	20:1 or more
Urine/plasma			
osmality ratio	<1:1	1:1-2	2:1 or more
Creatinine	<120	<120	45–100
			mmol/24 h
Sodium	>20	<10 mmol/l	—

11.1.1 Acute renal failure

Management of acute renal failure

Renal failure occurs when renal function is inadequate to control electrolyte and fluid balance. Acute renal failure progresses rapidly over a few hours or days and is characterized by rapid rises in:
Blood urea (normal range 2.6–6.5 mmol/l)
      creatinine (normal range 45–120 μmol/l)
      potassium (normal range 3.8–5 mmol/l).
Oliguria commonly occurs (500 ml urine in 24 hours), but acute renal failure can also be present with normal or increased urine volumes.

1 Identify, and if possible, eliminate the cause

Pre-renal failure

Urine characteristics: Normal sediment, urine osmolality >700, urine sodium <10 mmol/l.
Causes
Dehydration
Inadequate cardiac output

Blood urea can also rise rapidly in a hypercatabolic patient with normal or slightly impaired renal function.

11

Intrinsic renal failure

Urine characteristics: Sediment contains tubular cells, cell and granular casts. Urine osmolality is osmolar with plasma, urine sodium > 20 mmol/l.
Causes
Acute tubular necrosis (ATN)
Septicaemia
Prolonged hypovolaemic hypotension
Prolonged dehydration
Nephrotoxic drugs (may be antibiotics in hospital practice)
Hyperbilirubinaemia
Haemoglobin — mismatched blood transfusion
            — crush syndrome.

Other causes of intrinsic renal failure include glomerulonephritis, interstitial nephritis, pyelonephritis, and renal artery occlusion. These are rarely encountered as an acute situation and are strictly within the province of the nephrologist.

Post renal failure

Obstruction of the renal outflow tract. Blockage of a urinary catheter is a common, and easily remediable, cause.

2 Treatment

Pre-renal failure

In the management of pre-renal failure, from whatever cause, the early insertion of a Swan-Ganz catheter for measurement of pulmonary artery wedge pressure (PAWP) is an invaluable guide to left ventricular function, and may also be used to determine cardiac output by thermodilution. A central venous catheter must be inserted, as well as an arterial line if facilities are available.

Dehydration
Correct by replacement of fluid with normal saline initially. If available, colloid should be replaced in the form of plasma protein fraction (PPF), or blood until central venous pressure, arterial pressure and PAWP are normal. If oliguria persists, intrinsic renal failure must be considered.

Inadequate cardiac output
Cardiac output may be improved by infusion of an inotropic drug. Dopamine in a dose of 5–10 μg/kg/min is probably the drug of first choice, although isoprenaline, adrenaline or dobutamine may also be suitable. If these drugs become necessary, urgent removal to an intensive therapy unit is recommended.

Oliguria may also follow acute regurgitation of aortic or mitral valves and this may necessitate urgent surgery if ATN is to be avoided.

Intrinsic acute renal failure

Fluid balance
Basic replacement of 500 ml of crystalloid over 24 hours as normal saline or dextrose saline. This may have to be increased if the patient is pyrexial or is in a hot environment.

Replace other fluid losses from nasogastric tube, abdominal or chest drains. Replace the urine output hourly with a volume equal to the output of the previous hour.

The most useful index of fluid balance is accurate daily weighing of the patient.

Diuretics
Diuresis may follow an infusion of mannitol 20 g intravenously. If there is a normal CVP, this may be repeated once if there is no response.

The use of diuretics is controversial. In the opinion of some nephrologists, a single dose of frusemide 500 mg in 100 ml of normal saline intravenously over 1 hour is worth trying in acute

11

Renal failure diagnosis

oliguria as it may provoke a diuresis. In contrast, others believe that this is rarely effective in established intrinsic renal failure and the use of a large dose of frusemide may lead to further renal damage, with the added risk of ototoxicity.

Vasodilatation
Improvement in renal blood flow may follow general vasodilatation if the patient is vasoconstricted. This policy should be approached with caution as the possible fall in blood pressure may be difficult to reverse. If this is attempted, a short-term acting drug like phentolamine is the most suitable.

Dopamine induces renal vasodilatation in doses up to 5 μg/kg/min and this property together with the slight increase in cardiac output may induce a diuresis.

Electrolyte balance
Potassium must be measured frequently in the early stages of treatment. Plasma potassium can be controlled temporarily with:
Calcium resonium 15 g 6-hourly orally or 30 g rectally 12-hourly
Dextrose 25 g and insulin 10 units intravenously
Correction of acidosis by intravenous sodium bicarbonate

Other electrolytes, urea and creatinine should be measured daily and adjustments made to electrolyte intake according to the electrolyte content of fluid losses.

Nutrition
If the patient is not catabolic, a protein intake of 40 g/day with 2000–3000 calories may suffice. More commonly hypercatabolism will increase both protein and calorie requirements to much higher levels. A formula for estimation of nitrogen loss can be found in the section on nutrition (see Section 8) and in the hypercatabolic patient replacement of nitrogen and calories should be based on this if possible. In practice, fluid restrictions make this very difficult in most cases of renal failure in the intensive therapy unit.

If the patient is unable to eat, feeding should be by nasogastric route if possible. If not, intravenous feeding should be started as soon as possible. Calories can be provided from 50% glucose or fat, the choice of nitrogen source depends on how much is required. A convenient source is Vamin Glucose (Kabivitrum) which contains 9.4 g of nitrogen per litre (60 g of protein).

A more detailed account of this complex subject can be found in:
Hanson G.C. & Wright P.L. (1978) *The medical management of the critically ill.* Academic Press, London.
See especially pp.247–70, *The long term metabolic and nutritional management of the critically ill patient.*

Infection
Patients in renal failure are particularly susceptible to infection. Great care should be taken during the early stages in the handling of intravenous cannulae and central venous lines. A bladder catheter should only be used if it is really necessary.

Drugs
Many drugs, particularly antibiotics, must be given in reduced doses in renal failure. A detailed guide to drug dosage in renal failure can be found in:
British National Formulary, pp.9–14. The British Medical Association and The Pharmaceutical Society, London.

Dialysis
Dialysis should be considered if:
Blood urea is 40 mmol/l
Potassium is 6 mmol/l
There is evidence of fluid overload
There are uraemic symptoms, in particular, seizures, impending coma or vomiting
Uncontrollable metabolic acidosis develops.

50% of patients with acute renal failure die, usually of the various complications associated with the condition, even in experienced hands. If dialysis is required, it is best to transfer the patient to an intensive therapy unit experienced in dealing with renal problems. In

11

many cases acute renal failure can be treated by peritoneal dialysis without the need for a specialist nephrology unit. The contraindications to peritoneal dialysis are, widespread infection, recent abdominal surgery and uncontrolled hypercatabolism. If the patient exhibits some or all of these, and there is a high chance that haemodialysis may become necessary, the patient must be transferred to a specialist renal unit immediately.

SECTION 12
SI UNITS AND
CONVERSION TABLES

12

12.1 SI units

12.1.1 Basic units

In 1960 at the Conférence Générale des Poids et Mésures in France, the international units were formulated to standardize methods of denoting units and decimal points.

This was enlarged and developed into the Systeme International d'Unités (SI Units) and came into force in the United Kingdom on 1st October 1975.

The following list gives the basic SI units and their derivations, together with their recognised abbreviations. The letters *l, m, t* denote the basic concept of Length, Mass, Time from which the definitions of the derived units can be obtained.

e.g. Force can be represented as $\dfrac{\text{Mass x Length}}{\text{Time}^2}$

or Mass x Acceleration

Metre	m	unit of length (l)	
Kilogram	kg	unit of mass (m)	
Second	s	unit of time (t)	
Kelvin	K	unit of temperature	
Candela	cd	unit of light	
Decibel	db	unit of sound	1 decibel = 1/10 bel
Ampere	A	unit of electrical current	$\equiv 2 \times 10^{-7}$ Newton/metre
Hertz	Hz	unit of frequency per second	
Mole	mol	unit of amount of substance in grams	
Newton	N	unit of force	which gives 1 kilogram mass an acceleration of 1 metre per second^2 (mlt^{-2}) = Joule/metre
Pascal	Pa	unit of pressure	force per unit area ($ml^{-1}t^{-2}$) = 1 Newton/metre^2
Joule	J	unit of energy or work force through a distance ($ml^2 t^{-2}$) = 1 Newton metre	
Watt	W	unit of power	energy per second ($ml^2 t^{-3}$) = 1 Newton metre/second = Joule/second

SI Units

Coulomb	C	unit of quantity of electricity	$= 1$ Ampere second
Volt	V	unit of electrical potential	$= (ml^2 t^{-3} A^{-1}) = \dfrac{1 \text{ Watt}}{1 \text{ Ampere}}$
			$= \dfrac{1 \text{ Joule}}{1 \text{ Ampere. second}}$
Ohm	Ω	unit of electrical resistance	$= (ml^2 t^{-3} A^{-2})$
			$= \dfrac{1 \text{ Volt}}{1 \text{ Ampere}}$

12.1.2 SI fractions or multiples

10^{18}	exa	E		10^{-18}	atto	a
10^{15}	peta	P		10^{-15}	femto	f
10^{12}	tera	T		10^{-12}	pico	p
10^{9}	giga	G		10^{-9}	nano	n
10^{6}	mega	M		10^{-6}	micro	μ
10^{3}	kilo	k(K)		10^{-3}	milli	m
10^{1}	deca	da(D)		10^{-1}	deci	d

In this book we have, where possible, used the SI units. However, since the conversion depends on knowledge of the molecular weights, certain units cannot be in SI units. In these cases they remain in the old units.

Reference

Baron D.N. (1977) *Units, Symbols, and Abbreviations.* Royal Society of Medicine, London.

12.2 Conversion tables for physical units

12.2.1 Length

1 mm	= 0.0394 inches	1 inch (in)	= 25.4 mm
1 metre	= 1.0936 yards (yd)	1 foot (ft)	= 304.8 mm
1 km	= 0.6214 miles	1 yard (yd)	= 0.9144 m
1 Angstrom (Å)	= 10^{-1} nanometres (nm)	1 mile	= 1.6093 km
		1 nautical mile	= 1.852 km

12.2.2 Weight

1 g	= 0.0353 oz	1 ounce (oz)	= 0.4725 grains	
			= 0.02835 kg	
1 kg	= 2.2046 lb	1 pound (lb)	= 0.4536 kg	
1000 kg	= 0.9842 tons	1 ton	= 2240 lb	= 1016.06 kg
1 mg	= 0.0167 grains	1 grain	= 64.79 mg	
1 kg	= 0.1575 stones	1 stone	= 6.35 kg	
1 tonne (t)	= 1000 kg	1 cwt	= 112 lb	= 50.8 kg

12.2.3 Temperature

0 Kelvin (K)	= −273°C (Absolute zero)
273.15K	= 0°C = 32°F
373.16K	= 100°C = 212°F

$$°C = (°F - 32) \times 5/9$$
$$°F = (°C \times 9/5) + 32$$

°C	°F		°C	°F
30	86.0		36	96.8
31	87.8		37	98.6
32	89.6		38	100.4
33	91.4		39	102.2
34	93.2		40	104.0
35	95.0		41	105.8

12

12.2.4 Area

1 mm^2	= 0.00155 in^2	
1 m^2	= 10.764 ft^2	
1 m^2	= 1.1960 yd^2	
10 000 m^2	= 1 hectare	= 2.4711 acres
1 km^2	= 100 hectares	= 0.3861 miles^2
4046.86 m^3	= 1 acre	= 4840 yd^2
1 in^2	= 645.16 mm^2	
1 ft^2	= 144 in^2	= 0.0929 m^2
1 yd^2	= 9 ft^2	= 0.8361 m^2
1 mile^2	= 2.5899 km^2	

12.2.5 Volume

1 litre (l)	= 1 dm^3
1000 ml	= 0.03531 ft^3
1 m^3	= 1.3080 yd^3
1 l	= 0.22 gallons
1 ml	= 16.9 minims
1 l	= 1.76 pints
1 ml	= 0.282 fluid drachm
1 fluid drachm	= 3.55 ml
1 ml	= 0.0352 fluid oz
1 fluid oz	= 28.42 ml
1 in^3	= 16.387 cm^3
1 ft^3 = 1728 in^3	= 0.028317 m^3 = 28.317 litres
1 yd^3 = 27 ft^3	= 0.7646 m^3
1 gallon (UK)	= 4.546 l
1 minim	= 0.0592 ml
1 pint	= 0.5683 l = 20 fluid oz
1 teaspoon	= 4.5 ml ⎫
1 tablespoon	= 15 ml ⎬ approx.
1 teacup	= 120 ml ⎭
1 dessertspoon	= 8 ml ⎫
1 wine glass	= 60 ml ⎬ approx.
1 tumbler glass	= 240 ml ⎭

12.2.6 Speed

1 km/h = 0.2778 m/s   1 m/s = 3.6 km/h
1 knot = 1.852 km/h = 1.6 mph
1 km/h = 0.625 mph   1 mph = 1.6 km/h

12.2.7 Pressure

1 mmHg = 1.36 cmH$_2$O = 133.3 N/m^2 = 0.0194 psi
                        = 0.133 kPa
1 cmH$_2$O = 98.06 N/m^2 = 0.09806 kPa
1 psi   = 0.070 kg/cm^2 = 51.7 mmHg = 70.3 cmH$_2$O
          = 6894.76 N/m^2 = 6.895 kPa
1 atmosphere absolute = 760 mmHg = 14.7 psi = 29.9 inHg
                      = 1.03 kg/cm^2
          = 1.0133 x 10^5 N/m^2 = 101.33 kPa = 1035 cmH$_2$O
          = 1 bar = 1000 millibars
1 kPa   = 0.146 psi = 1.0 x 10^3 N/m^2

12.2.8 Work/energy

1 Joule (J) = 1 Nm
1 J   = 10^7 ergs = 0.239 calories (cal)
1 cal   = 4.1868 J
1 BTU   = 1055 J
1 kilowatt hour (kwh) = 3.6 x 10^6 J

12.2.9 Power

1 Watt   = 1 Newton metre/second = 1 J/s
1 horse power = 746 Watts = 550 foot pound/second = 746 Nm/s
1 metre kilogram/second = 9.81 Watts = 9.81 Nm/s

12

12.2.10 Force

1 Newton (N)   = 10^5 dynes
1 kilogram force (kgf) = 9.807 N
1 pound force (lbf)   = 4.44 N

12.3 Medical catheter gauge conversion table

SWG	Diam. in inches	Diam. in mm	English gauge	French Charriere
—	0.0156	0.390	—	1
26	0.018	0.457	—	—
—	0.019	0.500	00	—
25	0.020	0.508	—	—
24	0.022	0.559	—	—
23	0.024	0.610	—	—
—	0.026	0.660	—	2
22	0.028	0.711	—	—
21	0.032	0.813	—	—
20	0.036	0.914	—	—
—	0.039	1.00	0	3
19	0.040	1.02	—	—
18	0.048	1.22	—	—
17	0.056	1.42	—	4
—	0.059	1.50	1	—
16	0.064	1.62	—	—
—	0.066	1.66	—	5
15	0.072	1.82	—	—
—	0.079	2.00	2	6
14	0.080	2.03	—	—
13	0.092	2.33	—	7
—	0.098	2.50	3	—
12	0.104	2.64	—	—
—	0.105	2.66	—	8
11	0.116	2.95	—	—
—	0.118	3.00	4	9
10	0.128	3.25	—	—
—	0.131	3.33	—	10
—	0.138	3.50	5	—
9	0.144	3.66	—	11
—	0.157	4.00	6	12
8	0.160	4.06	—	—
—	0.170	4.33	—	13
7	0.176	4.47	—	—
—	0.177	4.50	7	—
—	0.183	4.66	—	14
6	0.192	4.87	—	—
—	0.197	5.00	8	15
—	0.210	5.33	—	16
5	0.212	5.38	—	—

SWG	Diam. in inches	Diam. in mm	English gauge	French Charriere
—	0.217	5.50	9	—
—	0.233	5.66	—	17
4	0.232	5.89	—	—
—	0.236	6.00	10	18
—	0.249	6.33	—	19
3	0.252	6.40	—	—
—	0.256	6.50	11	—
—	0.262	6.66	—	20
—	0.275	7.00	12	21
2	0.276	7.01	—	—
—	0.288	7.33	—	22
—	0.295	7.50	13	—
1	0.300	7.64	—	—
—	0.301	7.66	—	23
—	0.315	8.00	14	24
—	0.328	8.33	—	25
—	0.344	8.50	15	—
—	0.341	8.66	—	26
—	0.354	9.00	16	27
—	0.367	9.33	—	28
—	0.374	9.50	17	—
—	0.380	9.66	—	29
—	0.393	10.00	18	30
—	0.406	10.33	—	31
—	0.413	10.50	19	—
—	0.419	10.66	—	32
—	0.433	11.00	20	33
—	0.446	11.33	—	34
—	0.453	11.50	21	—
—	0.459	11.66	—	35
—	0.472	12.00	22	36
—	0.485	12.33	—	37
—	0.492	12.50	23	—
—	0.498	12.66	—	38
—	0.511	13.00	24	39

12

Benique gauge = 2 x French gauge: French = Charriere

SECTION 13
TOXICOLOGY

13.1 Introduction

A brief guide to therapeutic and toxic concentrations of some common drugs and other substances (National Poisons Unit, Guy's Hospital)

Notes:

1 All drug concentrations are measured in plasma except where otherwise specified

2 All drug concentrations are expressed in units of mg/l (equivalent to μg/ml) except where otherwise stated. SI units are not used yet in poisons centres

3 The data quoted in this guide is based on both the results obtained in this unit as well as reliable sources in the scientific literature

4 The concentrations quoted in this guide must be regarded as only approximations, which do not take into account certain variables which may modify individual drug response, i.e. weight, other medication, etc.

5 If in any doubt, the poison centres given below (with telephone numbers) will offer any doctor immediate information and guide to treatment. Calls are answered by trained information officers, and further advice can be obtained from the doctor on duty.

13.1.1 Poison centres

Guy's Hospital, London	01 407 7600
Cardiff	0222 569200
Edinburgh	031 229 2477
Dublin, Eire	Dublin 723355
Belfast	0232 240503

Other services also provide poisons information. The main ones are:

Leeds	0532 432799
Newcastle	0632 325131
Manchester	061 795 7000

13

13.2   Therapeutic and toxic blood levels

13.2.1 Drugs

Drug	Approximate peak level following a single therapeutic dose	'Therapeutic' range	'Toxic' levels usually greater than:	'Comatose' levels usually greater than:
Amiodarone		1.0–2.0	4.0	
Amitriptyline (+ nortriptyline metabolite	0.03	0.1–0.2	0.40	1.0
Amphetamine	0.05	0.1–3.0	3	—
Barbiturates				
Amylobarbitone	2	2–4	8	12
Barbitone	5	5–15	20	50
Butobarbitone	2	2–4	8	15
Cyclobarbitone	2	2–4	8	12
Heptabarbitone	2	2–4	8	12
Hexabarbitone	2	2–4	8	12
Pentobarbitone	2	2–4	8	12
Quinalbarbitone	2	2–4	8	10
Phenobarbitone	3	5–30	30	50
Bromide	5–25 (naturally occurring level)	—	500	3000
Carbamazepine	2.0	1.5–9	13	—
Chloral (as trichlorethanol)	10	10–50	50	100
Chloramphenicol		2–6	10	—
Chlordiazepoxide	1.0	3–7	8	13
Chlormethiazole	1.5	0.1–2.0	—	10
Chlorpromazine(free drug)	0.1	0.2–0.5	—	—

Desipramine	0.03	0.05–0.15	0.4	1.0
Dextropropoxyphene	0.2	0.2–0.8	1.0	3
Diazepam (+ desmethyl metabolite)	0.15	1–2	2	10
Digitoxin	5 ng/ml	14–30 ng/ml	30 ng/ml	—
Digoxin	0.5 ng/ml	1–2 ng/ml	3 ng/ml	—
Diphenhydramine	0.08	0.1–1.0	1.0	—
Disopyramide	3	2–5	8	—
Ethambutol	4	3–5	6	—
Ethanol (often expressed as mg/dl; can be converted by dividing by 10)	300	—	800 (legal UK driving limit) 1500 (clinically drunk)	3000
Ethchlorvynol	2	10–20	20	50
Ethosuximide	38	40–80	100	—
Fenfluramine (+ norfenfluramine metabolite)	0.06	0.1–1.5	0.2	0.7
Gentamicin	5	8–12	15	—
Glutethimide	2	2–4	8	15
Impramine (+ desipramine metabolite)	0.05	0.1–1.3	—	—
Indomethacin	—	0.7–1.3	—	—
Isoniazid	3	3–10	—	—
Lignocaine	1.0	2–5	5.0	—
Lithium	0.8 mEq/l	0.8–1.2 mEq/l	1.5 mEq/l	4 mEq/l

13

Therapeutic and toxic blood levels

Drug	Approximate peak level following a single therapeutic dose	'Therapeutic' range	'Toxic' levels usually greater than:	'Comatose' levels usually greater than:
Maprotiline	5	0.1–0.3	25	40
Meprobamate	0.05	5–10	—	—
Methadone	2	0.05–0.1	5	8
Methaqualone	—	2–4	40	—
Methsuximide		10–40	20	70
Methprylone	8.0	10–20	100	—
Methanol	—	—		
Morphine	0.07	0.05–0.5	0.25	—
Nortriptyline	0.04	0.05–0.15	0.25	1.0
Orphenadrine	0.15	0.1–0.2	0.5	5
Oxazepam	1.0	1–2	2	—
Paracetamol	15		200–300 (4 h post dose) 100–150 (12 h post date)	
Pethidine	0.5	0.2–0.8	2.0	—
Phenylbutazone		50–100	100	—
Phenytoin	5	7–20	20	50
Primidone (as phenobarbitone)	3	3–30	30	50
Procainamide	4	4–8	10	—
Propranolol	0.1	0.05–0.11	—	2.0
Protiptyline	0.02	0.1–0.3	0.5	1.0

Quinidine, Quinine	3	3–5	6	—
Salicylate	75	150–250	300	—
Sodium valproate	70	50–100	100	—
Theophylline	5	8–20	20	50
Verapamil	0.15	0.1–0.2	0.4	—
Warfarin	0.8	1–3	10	—

13

Therapeutic and toxic blood levels

13.2.2 Other substances

Carbon monoxide	HbCO (%)
Normal values	0.3–2.0
Tobacco smokers	1.0–10
Acute CO poisoning	20–30
Fatal CO poisoning	60–90

Cholinesterase	Normal values	(ΔpH units)
(Method of Michel modified by Larson)	Serum 0.5–1.2	Erythrocytes 0.6–1.0

13.2.3 Metals

Metal	Normal (μg/ l)	Hazardous (μg/ l)
Arsenic	< 20	> 50
Arsenic (urine)*	< 40	> 200
Arsenic (blood)	< 40	> 50
Arsenic (hair and nail)	< 1.5	> 2
Cadmium (blood and urine)	< 5	> 20
Copper (serum)	1–2 mg/l	
Lead (adult blood)	< 2.0 μmol/l	> 4.0 μmol/l
Lead (child blood)	> 1.5 μmol/l	> 3.0 μmol/l
Mercury (blood)	< 15	> 40
Mercury (urine)	< 20	> 100
Thallium (blood)	< 10	> 100
Thallium (urine)	< 20	> 200
Zinc (serum)	0.7–1.5 mg/l	

*Eating fish causes arsenic concentration to rise 100 μg/l

13.3 Guide to treatment of drug overdose

13.3.1 Introduction

The current mortality from all overdoses is less than 1%.
Respiratory complications are the principal cause of death,
principally from respiratory depression or aspiration of vomit. The
main treatment is therefore to maintain the airway and to provide
cardiovascular and respiratory support while the body eliminates the
poison.

Gastric emptying is considered useful in all salicylate overdoses
and in recent ingestion of other drugs where a potentially serious
amount has been taken. The patient should be conscious. In
semiconscious or unconscious patients, gastric lavage may be
considered, but endotracheal intubation must be performed first in
order to avoid the risk of inhalation of vomit. It is recommended that
300 ml of water at approximately 38°C be used repeatedly until a
clear lavage is achieved.

13.3.2 Forced alkaline diuresis

This is of value in:
1 Salicylate overdose
2 Phenobarbitone overdose (see section 7.8)

Suggested regimen for forced alkaline diuresis
500 ml 1.26% sodium bicarbonate   in rotation.
500 ml 5% dextrose   Monitor K^+ and CVP.
500 ml 0.9% saline   Urine pH should be >7.5

Give 1 litre in first hour then 500 ml hourly 10 ml of 10% Ca
gluconate t.d.s. $\pm$ frusemide 40–60 mg when necessary.

13

13.3.3 Forced acid diuresis

Although this is now seldom used it may be of value in poisoning
due to

Quinine   Fenfluramine
Phencyclidine   Pethidine
Amphetamine

Suggested regimen

5% Dextrose 500 ml + 1.5 g ammonium chloride
5% Dextrose 500 ml
Normal saline 500 ml
Infusion rate of 1 litre per hour. Urine pH is measured hourly and a
further 1.5 g of ammonium chloride added to the second 500 ml of
5% Dextrose if the urine pH exceeds 6.5.
   If sterile ammonium chloride is not available the urine can be
acidified by giving 2.5 g of ammonium chloride through a
nasogastric tube and repeating this if necessary.

Warning

Forced diuresis should not be undertaken lightly. If possible, the
patient should be in an intensive care unit. Hourly blood gas and
electrolyte estimations should be made, especially in the initial
stages. Particular attention should be paid to fluid balance and
potassium replacement.

13.3.4 Haemoperfusion

Charcoal haemoperfusion may be of use in cases of poisoning due
to:

Phenobarbitone   Trichlorethylene
All medium-acting barbiturates Paracetamol (late cases)
Glutethimide   Theophylline
Meprobamate

In the following circumstances haemoperfusion may be indicated.

1 Severe clinical intoxication
deepening coma ⎫
hypotension ⎪
hypothermia ⎬ resistant to treatment
hypoventilation ⎭
2 Deterioration in spite of treatment
3 Increasing plasma levels
4 Presence of complications (e.g. aspiration pneumonia).

13.3.5 Haemodialysis

Haemodialysis is of use with the following drugs and poisons:

Lithium	Bromide
Phenobarbitone	Salicylates
Alcohol, methyl and ethyl	Ethylene glycol

13

Index

211

213

Index